REVIEWS

Our hearts reach out to know there is something more than pain and suffering. We agonize for love to prevail in the storms that come our way. This is an amazing story of suffering redeemed by love that knows no time limits or boundaries. You will be staggered by the pain. You will be enthralled by the love. You will be surprised by the answers coming out of questions that have no answers. "Love Conquers Cancer" will take you on a journey from heartache to holiness. It will teach you how powerful reckless faith always is. This is a story of something more.

—Pastor Michael Simone
Spring Branch community church

I cried, I laughed, I was inspired. The pure courage and strong faith Andrea & Lenny have along the way is truly a page turner!

—Christi Fleck Privette
CEO of Two 17 Marketing

Through everything, all of it, Lenny & Andrea are still here, together. That's a true testament to love, marriage and commitment. Even for those without cancer, we could all learn a thing or two from reading their story.

—Aimee Thomas
Administrator, Software & Data Services

REVIEWS

When faced with life's challenges we all have a choice to succumb to the disease or fight with hope and perseverance. "Love Conquers Cancer" offers the deep truths about the fight and the courage to to see the miracles, peace, joy, and love through it all.

—Dawn Kroboth Martinez-
CEO His Healing Yoga

As I was discussing their trip to Mexico with Andrea on the phone, I asked her how long they were going to be there. If you could have heard the love and commitment that I heard in her voice when she said "oh honey, you know I'm not coming back without my man and you know we're not coming back until he's better", you would have teared up like I did. In that moment you wish someone loved you like Andrea Loves Lenny. This book is about faith, love and hope. It is their story. Read it and know that we can all make the world a better place if we just love.

—Dianna Good Sky,
Native American author of Warrior Spirit Rising

Love Conquers Cancer

DISCOVER HOPE AND
ALTERNATIVE HEALING ON
THE ROAD TO WELLNESS

Written by Andrea London
with Jack L. London

Resource Guide Included

Dedication

I want to first thank Jesus, our Savior and Lord. He truly is our Healer, provider, defender & Miracle Maker! We couldn't have gone through all of these battles and come out on the other side without Him!

To ALL of you who never gave up on us and our journey. You know who you are. Your prayers, endless support and encouragement mean the world to me and Lenny. I also want to thank our beautiful family (OUR ARMY).

I want to give a very special thank you to our beautiful children: Blake, Dylan, Diana and Jordan. You All have given so much to hold our family together! (To our babies, Jack & Jessica who are in Heaven, we can't wait to spend eternity with you two!)

To my hero. My hunk of a husband, Lenny.

Your love and belief in me helped me discover how to truly love and believe in myself. Your heart and your tenacity to live this life to the fullest and your determination to never give up hope inspired me to finally write our book.

And finally, to those of you whom we haven't met yet. Yes you. The overcomers. You who may be searching for answers in this crazy, upside-down world where sometimes life decides to throw several curve balls in a row. We have been praying for you.

Don't quit. You ARE an Overcomer!

This story is for you.

ACKNOWLEDGMENTS

There aren't enough words to truly express how we feel about ALL of the people who gave of themselves over the past 17 years and who continue to support our family to this day!

We wanted a section in the book just for you!

For everyone who has continually prayed for us and with us, we appreciate your diligence beyond! We know that there IS POWER in PRAYER!

For those of you who brought meals, cared for our kids, cared for our fur babies, took care of our home and yard, sent cards and gifts, made slideshows for our loved ones funerals, built Facebook pages and websites and set up fundraisers, designed our teams t-shirts, to the hundreds of amazing people who came together to support "Lenny's Day" to raise money for his alternative treatments, to the Beco family & the VB homes family and the many subcontractors who selflessly provided countless donations.

For those who paid for plane tickets and supplements and sent donations, for the amazing man who sent our family to Disney, for those of you who helped us with the entire "Operation Lenny" cannabis oil trip, visited us at hospitals and those who went to doctor appointments, to the amazing God's Girlz who listened, prayed and hosted garage sales for endless hours and selflessly donated the money to our family.

To Lenny's "Band Of Brothers" (you know who you are) for always coming together to rally behind our family.

To those of you who made hundreds of calls & texts to check in on us, and to the selfless family that loaned us the money to build our new home.

I know there's so much more but we truly wanted to mention ALL of these acts of love here and while we may not have everyone's name listed, We wanted to let you know that your acts of love remain in our hearts to this day.

To Pastor Simone and Gail who have been a constant support for our family, as well as Pastor Vinny Losciale & wife Jan, Pastor Kreg Vaughne & wife Faith, Pastors Chris & Alisha Mitchell and Pastors Archie & Tangie Callahan for taking the time to specifically cover our family in prayer.

To the United States Postal Service Headquarters prayer group for your constant prayers for Lenny & our family over the entire 17 years and to this day, we thank you!

To my mentors:

Pat and Carl Coleman (you literally helped change the course of my life!)

Toni Nolte for all those times of crying & praying in our cars, your endless encouragement and being such a prayer warrior!

Ryan & Shirona Anderson, the time you spent loving & encouraging us to never quit on our dreams, the prayers, the phone calls and texts, the gifts and the support you have constantly given our family have been nothing short of amazing!

To Diana for your endless hours designing, researching and adding your heart and passion to this project, your gifts are amazing.

To Blake, thank you for your encouragement and help for me to do the audio version & for sharing your gifts & talents so selflessly.

To my sister, Karen who consistently contributed ideas and reminded me to keep focused on "the why" behind this book.

To Dianna Good Sky who shared not only her encouragement but also her idea for the perfect title.

To Christi Fleck Privette and husband Keith, for their incredible marketing talent, being incredible cheerleaders for Lenny & I over the years and pushing us to do this.

To Susie & Tommy Hawthorne and Dawn & Mike Martinez for being brave enough to share their testimonies. Finally to the anonymous woman who encouraged me all those years ago while I was visiting CA to write this book & most recently to Natasha Haztlett who told me to "just write the darn book!"

CONTENTS

FOREWORD

CANCER—that one evil, nasty, word changes everything the minute your loved one is diagnosed. Confusion, shock, anger, an overwhelming sense of sadness. Then the questions. So many questions and not enough answers.

This book is written by my brother's wife, Andrea London, who has waged war against this evil disease, side-by-side with my youngest brother, Lenny, who was diagnosed with Non-Hodgkins Lymphoma over a decade ago.

Make no mistake, this is a very personal account of their life together. Andrea is very honest about the many challenges they have faced along the way, but more importantly, it provides detail and valuable insight into much needed information regarding alternative therapies for cancer.

Each individual who is facing a health crisis ultimately has to make the final decisions about their own care and treatment and that can be a lonely, terrifying place. It helps to have an advocate and if you are lucky enough an army, to help decipher the overwhelming information that will be coming your way. Lenny has an army and Andrea is his four-star general.

We have a very large family. When Lenny was diagnosed, we pitched in when and where we could with research, fundraising and doctor's appointments. But it was Andrea who spent countless hours on the internet, researching, reading books, making phone calls to doctors and clinics, reading recipes, and literally reaching out to anyone who may have a thought, an answer, or suggestion about Non-Hodgkins Lymphoma. Not to mention the numerous doctor's appointments, where she frequently challenged their professional opinions regarding treatment. She is constantly networking and providing Lenny with information, and together, they made (and continue to make) difficult, but informed decisions over and over again regarding his traditional and alternative cancer treatments. Tenacious does not begin to define this woman. Andrea's total devotion to my brother, her unwavering faith in God and her ability to remain positive even on the worst of days is remarkable. I love Andrea. She is my sister, she is my friend, and I truly believe she is the driving force that keeps our family positive, focused, and "London Strong."

Lenny. Honestly, I get choked up every time I try to convey my thoughts about my youngest brother. The minute you meet him you will instantly like him. He is friendly. He is funny. He's charming. He thinks he's hot, I think he's handsome. He is a kind, caring, and generous soul. He is loyal beyond belief to his friends and he loves his family unconditionally. I love my brother, and I am so proud of the man that he has grown up to be.

My intro mentions "the questions" and "not enough answers." To this day it is hard for me to wrap my head around why Lenny, of all people, was chosen. How could this nearly perfect husband, father, son, uncle, cousin, and brother be the one? No answer.

All I can tell you is that he has faced this monster head on, with the courage and strength of any warrior. His will to live, his incredible determination has inspired all of us.

This book is about Lenny and Andrea and their fight to love, to live, to hope.

As their battle continues, our family stands behind these two, amazingly, strong people. We will do what we always do in those times of need. We will pull together. We will rally and be there for each other. This time, it's for the love of Lenny.

Love always,
Karen

INTRODUCTION

The year my husband was diagnosed with Non-Hodgkins Lymphoma he joined an estimated 1.2 million other Americans[1] on a raging journey that not a single one of them asked to take. 1.2 million—diagnosed with cancer in a single year. That number does not even begin to include the countless millions already living with the disease, nor the countless millions who have been diagnosed since. For some the battle with cancer ends in victory and each year, for hundreds of thousands more, it does not. For Lenny and our family, the battle against cancer has raged for 17 years and continues still.

Ours is clearly not a new story. With the declaration of a single word, we joined the ranks of an army far larger than any the world has ever seen. As Lenny and I walked the path of diagnosis and treatment, something became increasingly unclear: if so many millions are facing the same enemy, how is it that we have not yet conquered it?

---

[1]   https://onlinelibrary.wiley.com/doi/10.3322/canjclin.51.1.15/pdf

This question launched us on a quest: to beat cancer no matter the method. Along the way, we realized that our goal was not just to see Lenny healed, but to also help others pursue and discover ways, both traditional and unconventional, to fight and conquer cancer. Lenny has undergone traditional treatment for Non-Hodgkins Lymphoma, but as there is no cure within the U.S. medical world for this type of cancer, he has also pursued and explored many types of alternative treatments. It was with the alternative medicine, and eventually treatment abroad that we experienced the greatest victories.

While ours has not always been a graceful fight, we have fought with a never-ending determination. It is this that we wish to share with you. This is not a tale of woe. It is not a journal chronicling a single family's grief, and pain, and the victories in between. This is a story about grit. It is a story about refusing to accept the status quo, the statistics, and above all else, refusing to give in to a disease that has ravaged the world for far too long.

This year, according to the National Cancer Institute, some 600,000 fathers, mothers, sons, daughters, aunts, or uncles will lose their battle against cancer.[2] Lenny and I will not allow another day to pass where this is our reality. We fight for healing and for a cure so that you or your loved one does not become part of this statistic.

Our hope and our prayer is that the steps we have already taken in pursuit of healing will not only provide encouragement, but be a resource for understanding that chemotherapy, radiation, and other traditional treatments are not the only option available. While these options do help eradicate some cancers, there is a world of research and effective alternative treatments that our

---

[2]   https://www.cancer.gov/about-cancer/understanding/statistics

society is only beginning to understand and accept. Within these pages we have chronicled every method of treatment we have tried over the past 17 years. Through trial and error, we have created a road map of best practices, diets, and alternative treatments. We have done the fieldwork so that others do not have to.

This is not just our story. This is a story for those who have gone before us, those whose lives ended far too early. This is for all who are still waging battle and those who are already walking in victory. Whether you are fighting cancer or any other disease or obstacle, this story is for you. May the pages that follow provide you with practical knowledge, indestructible determination, and absolute hope, for your story.

With lots of Love,
Andrea

CHAPTER ONE

The Diagnosis

Neither Lenny nor I needed to be told that his swollen lymph nodes were cancerous. He knew the moment he woke up from a high dose of anesthetic and saw that his body had been cut open and the lump removed. He had gone in for a biopsy; the fact that he had undergone surgery could only lead him to one conclusion. For me, the moment of realization came while I paced back and forth across the hospital waiting area, adding to the general anxiety of the room. As a door opened from the hallway, I looked up into the eyes of the approaching surgeon and felt a sinking in my gut, a desperation in my spirit. And I knew. I knew that the man I loved was about to face the most unexpected journey of his life. I also knew that I would face it with him.

When a loved one gets diagnosed with a chronic disease, it is difficult to describe the gamut of emotions that rushes through you. Fear. Dread. Disbelief. Anger. More disbelief. More anger. And then this undefinable emotion that launches you into a state of being that is strangely devoid of emotion: shock.

One thing I learned in the very early stages of Lenny's fight with cancer is that it does not discriminate.

We were married less than four months when we received the first diagnosis. Lenny had a swollen lymph node on his chin that would not go away, and he seemed to be in a perpetual state of exhaustion. Like a good married couple, I encouraged him to see a doctor and he ignored me. Out of desperation, I finally made an appointment for him.

Cancer is a unique disease to diagnose. It is, in fact, not one disease, but many. According to the National Cancer Institute, the rapid replication of cells that can occur anywhere in the body is the thread that ties each different cancer together.[3] Sometimes the cells multiply to form solid growths or tumors, other times the disease impacts the blood or prevents cells from naturally dying. Regardless, because of the multitude of ways cancer can impact the human body, it is not always easy to spot the disease for what it is.

The ear, nose and throat specialist that Lenny was encouraged to see had misdiagnosed a woman the prior year with a reactive

---

[3]   https://www.cancer.gov/about-cancer/understanding

lymph node. Not wanting to make the same mistake with Lenny, he prescribed a high-powered antibiotic for ten days. He then scheduled a biopsy surgery for the eleventh day, just in case the antibiotic didn't shrink the lymph node.

Eleven days later the lymph node was the same size. The plan was to take a biopsy of the lymph node with a pathologist standing by. If it was cancerous, they would remove the entire node right then, and if not, they would leave it for the time being.

Pacing in the hospital, after what seemed like days, but was surely only a few hours, I finally saw the doctor walking down the hallway toward me. As he approached to tell me what I already knew, every imaginable emotion flooded over me. *Why him? Why us? Why now?* The doctor looked somber as he recited the information. "I have taken out the lymph node and done the biopsy. The pathology showed lymphoma, we just don't know what kind or what stage it's in."

Somehow, hearing the truth was even more shocking than knowing it. I felt like I had been running at one hundred miles per hour and then suddenly hit a brick wall. I don't remember what the doctor said after that. I felt numb. My heart sank into my stomach and my stomach sank into my feet. *Lenny has cancer.* My brain tried to register the meaning of those words, but all I could register was the emotion that was threatening to pull me under. I mentally slapped myself in the face. *Hold yourself together,* I thought. A sense of helplessness flooded over me. Inwardly I fell apart and outwardly I did the only thing I knew to do: reassure this man in front of me that we would fight back.

I like to think that Lenny and I are a normal couple. We both met other people, started families, experienced heartache, and when it seemed that life would only ever be fraught with struggle, we found each other.

He had his career in construction and I had mine selling homes. We both had children that we were doing our best to raise with the values and strength—rather than the pain and hurt—that we had developed over the years. I had confidence and he had charm and a quiet wisdom. We both had a desire to live life with passion and enthusiasm, to love and be loved and experience the type of companionship that some say only comes along once in a lifetime.

We were married by the beach on September 1, 2001. My favorite aunt once said that rain on your wedding day is a sign that the bride and groom will shed a lot of tears in their marriage. When the rain starting falling the morning of our wedding, I didn't give it much thought other than to say a quick prayer. I had, after all, shed enough tears in my lifetime.

Throughout the ceremony, I remember my thoughts lingering on all of the possibility ahead of us. Lenny and I were bringing together the pieces of our past to create a new life and family. My two children and Lenny's son, together with us, would be the start of the London legacy, and sunshine or rain, there was hope in our future. As if to confirm my thoughts, as we joined our lives together that day, the rain stopped and the sun fought its way through the clouds.

Looking back, perhaps the rain was an omen that the years ahead would hold many more tears than we anticipated.

Or perhaps the weather that day was my reminder to not stand down, a foreshadowing that what we needed most was a passion to keep going, despite the obstacles.

Four months later, sitting in the hospital beside my husband, both of us grief-stricken and in shock, I imagined what this could mean for our lives. There were still many unanswered questions, facts and data we would collect over the next few weeks and months. In the moment, all I could really process is that the diagnosis was cancer, a feared and overpowering disease.

That day changed many things: our outlook, our plans, even our finances. One thing it did not change was who we are at the core. I believe it really only began a process of strengthening and challenging our best qualities, revealing and removing our worst. Of course, that is the wisdom of retrospect. That day I had no idea that the next 6,000 days would bring about the greatest challenge of our lives.

CHAPTER TWO

Watch and Wait

Being diagnosed with cancer is a series of events, rather than one heart-wrenching moment. It starts with an initial realization that cancer is present in the body, which for us was the day Lenny's lymph node was removed and we received the results of the biopsy. That was only the beginning. After his initial diagnosis, Lenny and I began a whirlwind journey of visits to different oncologists, seeking first, second and even third opinions.

Lenny, I have learned again and again, is a champion among human beings. I watched as he faced each event and obstacle of his diagnosis with a set determination. Prior to receiving a prognosis, he underwent a bone marrow biopsy to determine the type and stage of the Lymphoma he was fighting. I quickly discovered that observing your husband—or any loved one, for that matter—being stabbed with an 11-gauge needle is an emotional experience. Tears streamed down my face as I watched Lenny grit his teeth against the pain. My mind went wild with fear and frustration. *Why is this happening to him?* At the time, I did not receive an answer from God or anyone else.

Biopsies take time, and so a few days later we discovered the results. Lenny had Non-Hodgkins Small Cleaved Cell Lymphoma. At stage four, the oncologist determined that Lenny likely already had lymphoma for six or seven years.

I wondered how it was possible to live alongside a disease for so long and be completely unaware of its presence.

There are many different types of lymphatic cancers with one similarity: it affects the white blood cells that are key to helping your immune system ward off disease. Since lymph tissue is found throughout the body, lymphoma can start and spread from almost anywhere. The small cell lymphomas are slow-growing, or indolent, which often means the prognosis is to watch and wait. While large cell lymphomas are much more aggressive, they are also easier to treat and sometimes even curable. That was not the case with Lenny's diagnosis.[4]

We were told many things that day, but this is what I remember most: there is no cure, only treatment. Due to Lenny's young age, the oncologist recommended waiting

---

[4]   All lymphoma data found at: https://www.cancer.org/cancer/ non-hodgkin-lymphoma/about/types-of-non-hodgkin-lymphoma.html

before beginning treatments. Victims of the same type of Non-Hodgkins Lymphoma (NHL) could live for years, decades even. However, Lenny would likely run out of treatment options if he started too soon.

That particular oncologist was one of the best in our region, but he and I did not get along. His personality rubbed me the wrong way, our egos clashed, and his seemingly arrogant demeanor left me frustrated and protective. I learned to bite my tongue in his presence—at least in the beginning—since we needed his medical knowledge and advice in order to make the right decisions moving forward.

One thing the oncologist and I did agree on was the need for a second opinion. In fact, Lenny and I decided having a second and third opinion could only benefit us, and so we arranged to meet with experts both at Johns Hopkins Hospital in Baltimore, Maryland and Memorial Sloan Kettering Cancer Center in New York City. Both hospitals have some of the top Lymphoma specialists in the country, and we felt the odds of getting the best available options were in our favor.

Since the majority of Lenny's family lived in northern Virginia, they insisted on joining us in Maryland for our appointment with Johns Hopkins' top lymphoma oncologist. As we sat together in the hospital room discussing the results of Lenny's bone marrow biopsy, our family bombarded the doctor with questions. My hands were sweating and my heart was pounding as I tried to take notes on a giant legal pad. The prognosis was the same as we received in Virginia: watch and wait. Despite the fact that Lenny had 23 enlarged lymph nodes and cancer activity in his bone marrow, the oncologist agreed that conventional treatment should wait. At some point I stopped taking notes and just sat and listened.

As the appointment came to an end, the doctor looked over at me and asked if I had any questions. I said I only had one. "Please tell me that you have more than this. All the billions of dollars that are raised for cancer research in our country and all you have here is chemotherapy, radiation and a bone marrow transplant, and as a last resort?" I spoke with desperation. "Please tell me that Johns Hopkins has something all natural in the hopper that can cure this?"

His eyes lit up a bit and he began to explain their most recent clinical trial study on an ingredient found in rare plants and red wine called Resveratrol. This ingredient was thought to reverse the aging of cells and possibly even reverse cancer cells back to normal. I finally felt a modicum of hope return to me and I said, "Great! Let's get Lenny in this trial study." His expression changed again as he explained the study had just closed and that it would take approximately seven years to complete their findings.

Initially, in our excitement, my sister-in-law and I thought we could just get Lenny to begin drinking red wine. However, Lenny isn't a drinker and he would have to consume very large amounts of wine to have any positive effect on his cells. Of course, the effects of too much alcohol would counteract the resveratrol anyway. Once again our hope in anything the doctors had to offer was deferred.

As we drove home from Johns Hopkins, it was mostly quiet in the car. Lenny and I were both bewildered and overwhelmed. Suddenly Lenny asked me what I thought of it all, everything that we had been told so far. As for him, he did not feel comfortable with the prognosis of just sitting back and doing nothing while the cancer continued to spread through his body. I completely agreed.

We had already spent hours researching NHL and different methods of treatment, as well as natural options. I knew that a great place to start was with lifestyle changes. As we drove toward home that day, I said, "Babe, I think we should radically change your diet. Ramen noodles are not a food group. And we now know that cancer loves sugar, so you should also stop drinking Dr Pepper." In the moment, I didn't quite understand the significance of making different dietary choices. That would come with the wisdom of time. Our decision to pursue alternative treatments wasn't by mistake. It also wasn't a byproduct of distrust of the medical system—more like a moment of determination that there had to be more options available to us. Alternative medicine can be a scary pursuit; it has a stigma attached to it of being illogical, an option for people who distrust medicine and science and social standards. For us, alternative simply meant choice. If the oncologists had offered treatment options at the onset, I knew that we would have said yes to whatever was available to us. In fact, we would eventually choose traditional treatment when it became necessary.

I also knew in my heart that alternative methods could bring the healing we desired above all else.

For me, the choice to pursue health in whatever way possible was not unfamiliar. When my oldest son, Blake, was only five he began having seizures, and after taking him to several specialists, it was determined that he had epilepsy. However, I had this nagging feeling in my gut that the doctors were wrong.

Hewas prescribed a multitudeof medications, including Dilantin and Depakote, and after reading the side effects, I was hesitant to give him any of the available drugs for epilepsy. Instead, I began researching alternative treatments and we eventually ended up seeing a chiropractor.

The chiropractor took a completely different approach and after one look at his forehead, she noticed a scar. I explained that he had a serious fall the year before and then shortly after the fall, he had a bicycle accident because of "blacking out" which resulted in him receiving stitches both internally and externally on his head. Her response was immediate: she ordered x-rays for his neck and determined that his top three vertebrae were completely out of alignment. To my son, her explanation was simple: the injury to his neck was cutting off the "power" to his brain and she would adjust his back and neck to help turn the "power" back on.

Within six weeks of the alignment, all of his seizures had stopped. Within another eight weeks, I weaned him off all his medication (this was against the advice of the neurologist and not something I am recommending as a standard practice). The neurologist advised me that I was putting my son in danger and that his seizures would come back stronger than before. My son never had another seizure.

Thirteen years later, when he was hit by a car while riding his bike, he underwent a series of CT scans, and we discovered that he was born with one kidney. The drugs that were prescribed to him when he was five, which I refused to give him, are known to cause kidney and liver damage. I can only imagine what might have happened to his body if I had ignored the nagging in my gut.

With Lenny, the approach and the choice were the same. Some people believe we are here by mistake, that life on this planet is a byproduct of nature and natural occurrences. For me, life is significant, and everything has an intended purpose, a reason for being. Despite the prognosis, we knew that Lenny's life was valuable, worth every available option for healing, from prayer to chemo to resveratrol, and everything in between.

Something transitioned for us that day as we left behind the doctor and the prognosis from Johns Hopkins. The facts were clear enough; NHL with no cure and no immediate treatment. Watch and wait. However, a shift had occurred that would launch us into pursuing health at any cost—not just alternative treatments, but an alternative prognosis. One that included hope.

CHAPTER THREE

The Pursuit of Healing

Alternative, by definition, means "existing or functioning outside the established cultural, social, or economic system." Perhaps that is the best way to describe many things alternative: music, lifestyle, even alternative medicine. Another definition is, "one of two or more available possibilities." I like this definition because it expresses the one thing we often feel like we are lacking when it comes to fighting disease. It conveys our ability to choose.

Our appointment at Memorial Sloan Kettering was much like the previous two appointments. The prognosis was to watch and wait, and perhaps Lenny could eventually participate in future drug trials for NHL. With no traditional medical treatments available to him at that stage, it paved the way for us to launch an investigation into other treatment options that may not be readily accepted or advertised in the medical community.

We had already begun researching alternative treatments and after pursuing a local lead on an oncologist that didn't work out, we discovered a Wellness Center in Reno, Nevada. Our approach was simple: hold nothing back, pursue health and healing at any cost. Not knowing what else to do, or where else to turn, we made plans to fly to Reno and see what they had to offer.

I have learned many important lessons throughout this journey, one of those being the value in doing one's own research.

The medical field is riddled with controversial opinions and practices, treatments that are at the same time celebrated and criticized. In our divided world where opinion reigns, it is difficult to separate what is good and beneficial from what is not. Ultimately it comes down to not only finding trustworthy practitioners, but knowing within yourself how far you are willing to go in pursuit of health. The decision about treatment and what treatment to pursue is, and always will be, yours.

At the Reno clinic, we agreed to have the doctor perform several tests on Lenny that we had not heard of, including what is called a live blood cell analysis. While this type of analysis is considered controversial to this day, the potential of gaining knowledge about Lenny's condition far outweighed the risk that it might be an ineffective analysis. The tests that day showed evidence of the bacteria Borrelia burgdorferi. Lenny had a significant case of Lyme disease. Studies have linked Lyme disease to cancer, particularly NHL.[5] One of the struggles we faced with Lenny's diagnosis was the fact that he was young, healthy, fit and didn't particularly fit the criteria for Non- Hodgkins Lymphoma. The fact that his body was fighting Lyme disease was an incredible development on our search for understanding.

We were impressed by the results of the Reno clinic tests, but also concerned by the options, treatments and analyses the clinic was presenting to us. At the time, one option the clinic was promoting for cancer treatment was the issue of high doses of vitamin C by IV. Since we were both unfamiliar and uneducated about these treatments, Lenny and I approached the information we received that day with a level of caution.

During Lenny's final exam, the lead doctor asked if we had heard of a particular oncologist based out of Virginia. As we sat in his office discussing Lenny's results, he pulled one of his medical journals off the shelf and opened to a page referencing Dr. Vincent Speckhart, an oncologist who was also open to homeopathic treatment. I realized then that this doctor was not convinced that what the Reno clinic had to offer would benefit Lenny, but he obviously had confidence in Dr. Speckhart, enough to encourage us to meet with him.

Back at the airport, Lenny reminded me that we had tried making an appointment with Dr. Speckhart prior to discovering the Reno clinic. The doctor was in semi-retirement and not taking any new patients. I ignored him and in a moment of extreme determination, managed to locate Dr. Speckhart's

---

5   https://www.webmd.com/cancer/lymphoma/understanding-non-hodgkins-lymphoma-basics#1

home number. The doctor explained to us again that he was not taking new patients. He was in the middle of writing a book on his treatment methods and in partial retirement. I listened to him patiently and then I begged him to see Lenny. I explained our situation, the Reno clinic, our goal to get Lenny healed by whatever method was available. I begged and he finally conceded.

Dr. Speckhart came with his own history of controversy, much like any medical doctor seeking to understand alternative ways to treat disease. His methods were unique, sometimes criticized, but he sought to partner alternative options with standard medical treatments. At one point, he stood before a Congressional committee to defend his methods and described his reasoning for pursuing complementary medicine: "After 13 years of using FDA- approved chemotherapy protocols, I concluded that such therapies were extremely toxic, poorly tolerated, and not effective in prolonging survival in most solid tumors of adults. In 1983, my patients began to request therapies other than chemotherapy. I agreed, and without even knowing it, I became an 'alternative practitioner' and was red-flagged by opponents of this form of therapy."[6] When we walked into Dr Speckhart's office, an old renovated home, I was a bit apprehensive due to the condition and the fact that we were the only other people in the office.

However, when the doctor walked out to greet us and we made eye contact and shook hands, I had an overwhelming sense of peace that he was going to help Lenny. Once in his office, one

---

6   https://articles.mercola.com/sites/articles/archive/2011/08/06/
     why-we-dont-have-a-cure-for-cancer-yet-or-do-we.aspx or http://www.
     healingpathwaysmedical.com/docs/chemotherapy-ineffectiveness.pdf

of the first things he asked us was if we ascribed to any particular faith, and we both answered that we were believers in God. He went on to tell us that 80% of getting well was believing. He explained his choice to pursue alternatives to conventional medicine after thirty years of practicing as a physician. Many of his former patients experienced horrible side effects to chemotherapy and he knew that there had to be a better way to heal people of cancer.

One of his methods of testing was the use of electronic frequencies and acupuncture points to determine what was wrong in the body. While this isn't a conventional way to diagnose an issue, his years of experience showed him that it was a useful method to discover the root cause of cancer in the body, helping provide better understanding of where to begin in order to eliminate the disease.

Without much further explanation, Dr. Speckhart connected several wires and handed what looked like two probes to Lenny. Before I realized what was happening, a printer connected to the wires began to spit out sheet after sheet of paper. Each sheet contained a reading that identified various problems in Lenny's body, including the presence of Lyme disease—confirming the analysis from Reno—and several inherited issues.

After reading the results of the electronic frequency test, Dr. Speckhart began mixing small bottles of alcohol, placing them on this attached machine that would add specific frequencies to the liquid. He carefully labeled each bottle with instructions on how to administer them and how many to take each day. We left that first visit with half a dozen bottles and instructions to come back in thirty days.

At this point, our doubt began to outweigh our hope and trust in this alternative approach. The methods were far-fetched, at best, and I looked at the little bottles of alcohol with a new-found skepticism. Any quick internet search would produce a number of critical responses to Dr. Speckhart's work, enough to make one pause. But then something strange happened. Lenny called his mother and asked if she had been exposed to tuberculosis and some other toxins that had been present in his electro-frequency results. She became instantly emotional and asked Lenny how he knew. Her shock and emotion were enough of a response for us to know the truth of the test results. Doubt or no doubt, the results proved valid, and hopefully the treatment would as well.

After about five months and several visits with Dr. Speckhart, the frequency test no longer produced any negative readings and Lenny was able to eliminate his use of the alcohol drops. Throughout this treatment, we had also initiated a healthier diet and a regimen of powerful supplements in an attempt to remove toxins from the body as well as get Lenny's immune system in good working order. Dr. Speckhart recommended we invest in a far infrared sauna, as well. The infrared light of the sauna helps increase heart rate and release toxins through sweat—similar benefits as vigorous exercise. We added the sauna to our list of treatments, along with diet, exercise and supplements.

Lenny was due to have scans done by our original oncologist shortly after he finished his round of alternative treatments. We were prepared to see improvement, expected it, in fact. The scan revealed that all 23 lymph nodes had returned to their normal size, only one node remained slightly enlarged at .5 centimeters. We were thrilled with the positive report. We were also completely shocked when the oncologist refused to acknowledge the improvement, and instead focused on the one lymph node that was still enlarged.

I was furious. Dr. Speckhart had warned us of this, noting that in his experience the conventional physicians would not often acknowledge the alternative methods as having any value or relevance. Despite the foreknowledge that this might be the case, I still struggled to see how anyone could ignore the truth: Lenny's body was responding to natural treatment and the proof was in the scan.

Conventional methods dictated that Lenny could not be classified as in remission due to the presence of the one slightly enlarged lymph node. Despite our excitement at the improvement in Lenny's body, the response from the oncologist was discouraging. After taking a few days to process the news, Lenny and I decided it was time to make some changes. We requested that the physician put in writing the positive results of the scan, noting the changes since the previous diagnosis. We then decided to find a new oncologist.

With a disease like cancer, or any chronic illness that requires extensive medical attention, finding the right physician is like finding the right therapist or mentor. Trust is certainly an important factor, as is worldview and frame of mind.

When healing is the goal, regardless of method, having care and support from the medical world is absolutely priceless. So we discovered.

Dr. Alberico proved to be the complete opposite of our previous oncologist in both attitude and disposition. Not only did he come highly recommended, but his approach was open and accessible. He carried both empathy and confidence, which in turn gave us confidence. At our first appointment he shared that, "All medicine is an educated guess." While he did not know much about the alternative treatments available, he did not disagree with them. Of our pursuit of different options, he simply acknowledged that we had to do what we felt was best for Lenny. "God is in control," he stated. And I knew that he would walk this journey alongside us.

After Reno and Dr. Speckhart, and the lifestyle changes that came with the natural treatments, we felt confident that we were on the right path. Alternative worked for us, and we would continue to pursue health in this way. Finding Dr. Alberico solidified Lenny's desire for a complementary approach. He would carry on with his regular scans and check ups with the oncologist while still continuing with natural treatments and lifestyle changes. We settled into our new reality and new routine with greater confidence and assurance than at the outset. It ultimately came down to choice. If there was an option available that would lead to healing, we would choose it.

CHAPTER FOUR

Jack and Jessica

We like to believe that when bad things happen the world completely stops. In our hearts, we imagine that in the midst of chaos or devastation there is a moment of pause—like in the eye of a storm—when we'll experience revelation on how to proceed, peace and confidence in our path, and perhaps even a moment of healing from what came before. Life doesn't stop; it doesn't even slow. It is not sympathetic to our cause in the way that we must learn to be. Instead, life is a train that keeps moving at such a pace we know we will never be able to catch up with it. And then we discover we've been on it all along.

When Lenny was first diagnosed with NHL, I already felt like life had left me far behind. In our tiny beach cottage was a room I had lovingly decorated and prepared for the arrival of our first child together. Our son was due to arrive in the new year, and while my body did not take well to the pregnancy, I was elated to be adding to our family.

At 26.5 weeks, Lenny woke me in the middle of the night to the sight of water and blood-soaked sheets. Neither of us were prepared for this unexplainable tangent from normal life. Fear mixed with confusion as I tried to comprehend what this meant. After Lenny rushed me to the hospital, I heard one of the nurses say, "We can save the baby," and I was able to breathe again.

Within a few hours, however, I was rushed to a different hospital, one with a high risk pregnancy unit, and the fear and confusion quickly transitioned to panic. When the doctor told me that they couldn't save the baby, I argued with him. Surely he was wrong. And if he wasn't, surely I would die. I thought perhaps I wanted to.

Someone, somewhere started me on an IV of medication to help speed my labor, and through those next nine hours I pushed, and pleaded for a miracle. Our baby boy was born that evening, but he never took his first breath. His name was Jack.

The pain of loss came in waves, each carrying an accusation. I failed my husband. I was supposed to give him a son and I have given him nothing. I ate the wrong thing, didn't exercise enough, I somehow did something deserving of this loss. How could it be anything but my fault?

Loss has a way of tormenting us, but usually, with time, the torment starts to fade. Even before it fades, we often learn to ignore the barrage of accusation and move forward with our lives, choosing to forgive ourselves, even if we've done nothing that needs forgiveness. While this was my philosophy, allowing time and God to heal my wounds, it was not to be my reality. At least not yet.

Baby Jack was cremated and his ashes placed in an urn carrying an inscription of Matthew 19:14. "Jesus said, 'Let the little children come to me, and do not hinder them, for the kingdom of heaven belongs to such as these.'" The verse comforted me, and so did the presence of his little urn on our bedroom dresser. At least for a time.

A few short months later found us sitting in an oncologist's office facing an entirely new obstacle. Instead of taking time to mourn our loss, we were suddenly faced with the challenge of fighting for life. Lenny's life. The world hadn't stopped for baby Jack, and neither could we.

I've always faced life with a certain sense of passion— some might call it intensity, but I like to think of it as an unwillingness to give up. After losing Jack, my emotional state was fragile, at best, but with my husband's well-being in question, my drive to find a solution overtook my need to pause and heal. That began our whirlwind experience of seeking opinions from Johns Hopkins and Sloan Kettering, and eventually the alternative treatments from the Reno clinic and Dr. Speckhart. Those first few months of life post-diagnosis were a test in both strength and mental health.

Everyone has their unique method of facing life's challenges. Some find stability in staying active or in being around others, or by practicing meditation or prayer. I found my stability in worship. I began my spiritual journey when I was eleven, in a beautiful chapel I attended a few times with my mom when I was young. It was a Sunday in May, Mother's Day that year, when the pastor gave the invitation to accept Jesus as our savior, and I practically ran down the aisle to meet this savior, my mom right beside me.

While Lenny holds the same beliefs, our expression of faith is unique to each of us. He was raised without much religious influence, but he could not help but see the world around him as a byproduct of something beyond his own understanding.

As he grew older, his observations and questions led to a belief in God. Lenny has always been very quiet about his faith and jokingly says that I have enough to say about it for the both of us. Lenny's character, his kindness and patience, however, are more an expression of God's love than any words or religious act.

Those first few months it was moments of quiet, of prayer and worship that were my fortitude.

Despite the emotional turmoil we had already sustained with Jack's loss, we faced every appointment and diagnosis with a conviction that our lives have purpose and that God is in the midst of that purpose.

Outwardly, I fought hard to do what needed to be done. I sold houses, I made appointments with oncologists, and I took care of our three kids. Inwardly I was struggling. The conviction and the faith existed alongside an enormous amount of pain.

Life, in its usual fashion, kept moving forward. Lenny was responding to the alternative treatments that Dr. Speckhart offered, and I was pregnant, this time with a little girl. I was apprehensive about getting too excited until I knew I was going to be able to carry her to full term, and so we cautiously went through each day and every visit to the doctor. Due to my previous pregnancy, the physicians were careful, but there was no plan in place for what would happen if my water broke between visits.

Just shy of 20 weeks, my water broke at home and I ended up at the hospital for an emergency D&C due to miscarriage. It was Mother's Day weekend. Grief felt surreal this time around. It was as though I never truly became emotionally attached to our daughter, and I handled the loss with seeming indifference. Lenny, on the other hand, never truly grieved losing baby Jack and so the loss of our daughter tore him apart. He wanted to see her and hold her. I simply felt like a failure as a wife and a mother.

D&C is normally an outpatient procedure, so before leaving the hospital that day, I told the administration to please call me when pictures of our daughter were ready to be picked up. The hospital takes care to provide photos of all the babies born there. With Jack, the pictures showed up unexpectedly in the mail. I was sure I wouldn't be able to handle that again. Perhaps I didn't feel indifferent after all.

Jessica's ashes joined those of her brother in the little urn marked with the verse from Matthew. We did our best to properly grieve, but like before, life seemed to have other plans. There were too many things to accomplish, bills to pay, doctor's appointments to schedule, and three other kids to raise. Thankfully, Lenny's next scans showed the reduction in all but one of his lymph nodes and we finally had something to celebrate.

Life does not slow down in the midst of chaos. Sometimes, we have to slow ourselves down. I didn't know that at the time.

Rather than stop to breathe and let myself be in the moment, feel the pain and let it wash away, I ran head first into the problems thinking I could solve them all.

Or at least I could try. "Why are you running a hundred miles per hour?" Lenny would ask, "Slow down." If life wouldn't slow down, how could I?

It would be some time before I learned how to heal and care for myself.

The journey of faith or belief of any kind takes time, years even—some would say a lifetime.

While I am still learning what it looks like to live from the faith that I felt so compelled toward as a child, that worldview and belief were the sustaining force behind the past two decades of my life. Eventually it would also be a source of healing.

At that time, however, my focus was on keeping up with everything in front of me. Life was moving fast forward and I was swept away with its incessant forward motion. Lenny and I both were overcome with our drive to see him healed. Life doesn't even stop for cancer, I discovered. We worked, we fought disease, we did our best to love our family, and we lived. And life just kept right on moving.

CHAPTER FIVE

The Importance of Living

Doctors often use what is called the International Prognostic Index to determine an estimated life expectancy for NHL patients. The index looks at factors such as the patient's age, stage of the lymphoma, and how much and where the lymphoma is in the body.[7] For slower growing—or indolent—lymphomas, the index measurements are slightly different, but the overall outcome is still the same. Patients are categorized into a risk group, each of which has a 5 and 10 year percentage rate of survival. These are only estimates, the doctors assure you, and estimates based off of the previous decade's patients and therefore based off of the treatment options that were available ten years ago.

---

[7] https://www.cancer.org/cancer/non-hodgkin-lymphoma/ detection-diagnosis-staging/factors-prognosis.html

Lenny was given seven to nine years to live. Since treatment options really had not changed much in the previous several decades, it was this extended timeline and Lenny's age that determined the prognosis of watching and waiting. For Lenny, however, he was being asked to watch and wait as he slowly reached an expiration date.

Fully comprehending and coming to terms with your own mortality is a process as original as the individual experiencing it. Journeying through life's bigger questions has as much to do with perspective as it does personal belief. It is, however, universally overwhelming. When first faced with an abbreviated life expectancy, Lenny hounded the oncologist with questions. "What is Lymphoma?" he asked. "How do you get it? What eventually kills you?" He didn't receive any solid answers.

Internalizing his fear and instead focusing on his disbelief, Lenny faced the next hurdle of passing this information on to his family. On the drive to Northern Virginia, he informed me that he would do the talking and that I should try not to cry. "I will tell my family, because you will get emotional," he stated. Tears are a fairly standard response to life-changing news, however, and it turns out he didn't need to worry about me after all. His voice broke with emotion as he shared the results of his scans with his family and they in turn wept. That is, I think, what love looks like.

Family is the first line of defense, the very first support system available to lean on in times of need.

At home, we had a family of three, sometimes five, in the little three bedroom beach cottage that Lenny bought before we married. My daughter lived with us full time, while each of our two sons came and went on weekends and holidays. This was our sanctuary, our little haven from the storm. The kids were old enough to understand that Lenny was fighting for his life, but young enough to not quite comprehend the full extent of that prognosis. I knew their young minds were absorbing the depth of our battle at some level, and so we did our best to make our home feel safe and normal. Eventually, Lenny's father joined our little community as well. This was not a thrilling transition for me, at first. Family, your greatest support, can also be your greatest weakness. I almost threw the towel in after my father-in-law's first week with us. We fought, I complained to Lenny, and eventually, over time, love prevailed. He was family, after all, and I could see how much his presence was a support to Lenny.

While family is the first line of defense in a struggle, community is most certainly the second. As humans we don't always do everything right the first time, but we wouldn't get very far without one another. Support comes in many different forms and has many different meanings. Encouragement, relief, assistance, strength—all are varieties of support, whether financial or emotional. When we lost Jack and then Jessica, people brought food and flowers, letting us know that we were not mourning alone. Community is a beautiful gift.

When Lenny was first diagnosed, our community and family were sometimes unsure of how to help us, and we were unsure of how to receive. In the overwhelming moments, the well-meaning questions became burdensome. "What can we do?" became a hindrance more than a help, forcing me to delegate need and designate tasks. I couldn't even communicate my needs, let alone delegate them to someone else.

Lenny's family rallied around us during this time and his sister, Karen, organized a fundraiser to help pay for the alternative treatments. "Lenny's Day" was a huge success. There was a band, food, prizes and a few hundred people who lovingly came to support Lenny and donate toward the treatments. We were overwhelmed with goodness, and strangely, I was also overcome with grief.

It was not the ideal time to grieve. The day was about Lenny; it was his family's way of showing their love for him. We were surrounded by old friends and new ones, community we had built together as a couple, alongside friends Lenny had known since childhood. In the middle of all that love and support, all I could focus on was loss. The presence of Lenny's first wife seemed to press the wound of my recent miscarriage, emphasizing my insufficiencies as a wife and mother. All around me people were celebrating and sharing their love, and all I knew was my own failure. Beneath it all was the fear of the unknown that Lenny and I had each so successfully ignored; the fear of what might happen to Lenny if treatment didn't work.

Grace is a precious thing, something we must extend to ourselves as much as to those around us.

After my emotional breakdown at Lenny's fundraiser, I still did not know what it was we needed or how to ask for help. I did know that I was broken, and Lenny was sick, and we were on a mission that left little room for facing what any of that meant for us emotionally.

It was in the most unexpected moment that we received the help we didn't know we needed. We had faced the reality of Lenny's diagnosis, but had not fully processed the meaning of it. In a single question, Lenny's friend helped him face the truth. "If God calls you home to heaven sooner rather than later, what is one thing you have to do before you go?" he asked. It is a simple thought, innocent really, but it begs an even more profound question.

Now that you might die, how will you choose to live?

Lenny's response was as pure and honest as the question. If there was one thing he wanted, it was to spend time with his son and take him to Disney. Lenny had already decided how he would live in the face of the unknown: sharing every moment with those he loved. A few weeks later we received an all-expense paid trip to Disney World. Lenny's friend shared their conversation with another friend, a stranger to us, who made it his mission to give Lenny his wish. Again, the generosity of community washed over us. How is it that a complete stranger would be so willing to pour into our lives? My daughter and I joined Lenny and his son on what proved to be one of our most memorable family vacations. We laughed together, enjoyed performances and rides, and the kids experienced their first taste of Disney magic. Years later, my daughter would tell me that for her, the trip was just a normal part of life, something all families do together. It was not weighed down by the heaviness of cancer, and for that I am forever grateful.

Lenny and I learned several things in that season, including how to enjoy the moment and the value of generosity. Most importantly, despite the unknown, we learned to live. Life was still moving at a momentous pace, and there would continue to be doctor appointments and treatments to pursue. Our babies were still gone, and nothing was certain, but when we looked at what we did have, everything looked more hopeful. Lenny had his good report of reduced lymph nodes, our kids were healthy and happy, and we would keep on living.

In the spirit of moving on with life, we decided that our little beach cottage was beginning to feel overcrowded. Lenny and I were both prospering at our jobs and we made the decision to purchase property near some friends of ours and build our own home. The next season was a peaceful one. We designed our dream home and enjoyed the nearness of friends and family. I found out I was pregnant again, and somehow I knew the baby would be healthy, and that he would be a boy.

A year earlier I met a young OBGYN at an open house. Between showing her the property, we talked about life and loss, and eventually I shared about my two previous pregnancies. In a strange moment of vulnerability, I shared that I thought the loss of our babies could have been prevented with better prenatal care. She listened with compassion and then gave me her contact information. "Call me when you become pregnant again," she said, "and I will deliver your baby!" At the time I was certain we would not be having any more children, and I told her as much. Still, I set her card aside rather than throwing it away.

After realizing I was pregnant, I found the business card from the year before and made an appointment with Dr. Thibodeau.

As with the previous two pregnancies, I was very sick, but Dr. Thibodeau was diligent and precautionary in her approach. She put me on bed rest at 20 weeks and put in two stitches in my cervix to keep the water in the uterus. I am an overachiever, and bed rest grated against my need to get things done. To combat my unrest, I took up crochet and, to Lenny's dismay, online shopping. The kids helped around the house and Lenny discovered Walmart and the glory of getting all the shopping done in one location. Somehow we made it to 40.5 weeks. The cerclage was removed, and after a steady round of walking, a full spaghetti dinner and some strawberry daiquiri, Jordan Leonard London decided to join us. He was perfect and he was healthy.

Even though life expectancy is just an estimate, it is that looming reminder that everything could end sooner than you imagine. That alone is a paralyzing reality. We still didn't have any solid answers to Lenny's questions— how long he would live, how best to fight the disease. We only knew that the beauty of living is what keeps us going. Our children were a constant demonstration of what that looks like. The pure delight in their eyes at Disney, the joy of meeting their new brother, the adventure of building a home—these were the things that helped us forward.

New life has a way of making every worry and fear seem meaningless, even powerless.

Jordan was our renewed promise that the only way to possibly move forward in life was to face it head on, with as much joy and determination as possible. We would still combat fear, and the unknown would always be steadily before us, but those were nothing compared to what we had been given. It is in the presence of family, community, love and generosity, that we are reminded to live.

CHAPTER SIX

Cancer and Conventional Medicine

Giving and awareness are a huge part of our society's fight against cancer. Almost every month of the year is dedicated to the awareness of a specific type of cancer, or cancer prevention, control or research. Over a billion dollars are donated each year to cancer research through fundraising events, while the United States government designates just over $5 billion[8] and pharmaceutical companies spend many billions more. Since President Nixon passed the National Cancer Act of 1971, over $500 billion has gone into the war on cancer. Progress has been made, as evidenced in the longer life expectancy, on average, for patients diagnosed with cancer.

---

[8]   https://www.cancer.gov/about-nci/budget/fact-book/data/research-funding

However, the number of people being diagnosed has also dramatically increased over the last half century. The arguments go both ways, some defending the value of research being done and others challenging its slow progress.

We became increasingly aware of these trends the further we researched treatment options for NHL. Every time Lenny stopped at a 7-Eleven, his eye would catch the little donation cups by the register inviting customers to give their spare change to help fight cancer. He would walk away wondering where that money was being spent. Would it go toward finding a cause, perhaps preventing some of the many different types of cancer? Or was it going to formulate more drugs that would be too expensive or too dangerous for the cancer patients who need them most?

On the other side of this expensive trend is not the money spent on research, but on purchasing the cancer treatment medicines that are currently available.

In 2017, the worldwide total expense on cancer treatment drugs exceeded $130 billion.

That number is expected to grow to $200 billion by 2022. In that same time period, spending on cancer treatment drugs in the U.S. alone could reach $100 billion annually.[9] Those numbers don't even begin to cover the expenses on medical

---

[9]   https://www.iqvia.com/institute/reports/global-oncology- trends-2018

appointments, scans, and all of the smaller costs of living with cancer that add up for every family and patient diagnosed.

On a personal level, Lenny and I were aware that despite the money being funded for research, the options available for NHL patients were limited. Not only were they limited, but should they become necessary, they were also extraordinarily expensive and in many cases, ineffective. Having already undergone the alternative frequency treatments, which were not covered by insurance, we were equally aware that fighting this disease in any way would be costly.

Three years into our journey we faced this reality in an entirely new way. Lenny started complaining about pain in his neck and our chiropractor, who had been regularly adjusting him, refused to touch him again until he got an MRI. He reluctantly agreed. Up until that point, he hadn't experienced any other symptoms of NHL, and we were continuing the diet, sauna and supplement regimen suggested by Dr. Speckhart.

A few days after the MRI, Lenny's sister and brother-in-law came to visit us for the holidays. Just as they arrived at our house, the doctor called with the results from the scan. Without warning, everything shifted. Lenny was told to go to the Virginia Beach Hospital and check in through the emergency room. They would be expecting him.

That familiar feeling in the pit of my stomach returned as we prepared to leave for the hospital. Lenny's sister and her husband agreed to stay with the kids and we rushed out the door. In the car Lenny asked me if I thought it was the cancer again, and I reassured him that it wasn't. I thought for sure lymphoma couldn't show up in the neck and back, that it had to be something else like a strain or fracture from working out. As much as I tried to convince myself otherwise, I knew in my heart that something was wrong.

We checked Lenny in to the ER and the process went by very quickly since they were expecting him. Once he was assigned a room, a young doctor joined us to explain what was happening. There was a mass in Lenny's spine and he strongly recommended that they begin a round of radiation and steroids immediately. I stared at the doctor, and all I could think about was how young he looked. Too young to be practicing medicine, I was sure. Or at least, too young to provide a correct diagnosis.

In a moment of disbelief, I told him to go wake up his boss or a more experienced doctor. I suggested he get an oncologist, while he was at it, someone who would have more knowledge about the situation. Less than thirty minutes later, and older doctor found us in the room and at my urging, brought us the MRI films to explain what was happening to Lenny's body. He pointed out a very large mass wrapped around Lenny's spinal cord. "If we don't begin shrinking this mass tonight," he said, "your husband could be paralyzed by morning." We found his explanation of events to be significantly more convincing, and so we agreed that Lenny should start the radiation and steroid treatments immediately.

The next six months consisted of 20 rounds of radiation, six rounds of intravenous chemotherapy and four rounds of intrathecal chemotherapy—the injection of drugs directly into the spinal column. These treatments were topped off with prednisone, which Lenny hated the most. While none of it was pleasant, he complained that the steroids made him moody and bloated, and due to an insatiable hunger, he gained 40 pounds within the first few months.

I went with him to every treatment, not only to be his designated driver, but to provide whatever support I could during the process. The first round of chemotherapy took several hours for each treatment, first requiring a blood test and then, if his blood count, liver and kidneys checked out, a round of R-CHOP would be administered intravenously. This particular cocktail was made up of five different cancer-killing drugs. At the time, we refused to read about common side effects of the treatment.

We knew that the drugs were essentially killing the rapidly reproducing cells, but they were also poisoning Lenny's body.

After each round of chemotherapy, we would return home and Lenny would disappear to the bedroom to sleep for a day or two. He called it the "hurricane effect" and said it felt as if a hurricane was ripping through his insides. He barely ate during those times and I had to plead with him to stay hydrated. While the chemo can lower blood counts, it also compromises the immune system and puts patients at risk for infection. I filled Lenny with food and water in an attempt to keep him as healthy as possible.

The intrathecal chemotherapy was probably the most difficult part of the process, both for Lenny and for me. The drugs were inserted into his spinal cavity to kill any cancer cells that may have leaked into the spinal fluid. He was supposed to complete six rounds of treatment, but on the fourth round the doctor hit Lenny's sciatic nerve with the needle. Lenny yelled out to stop the treatment, saying it felt like a land mine had just exploded inside his body. I sat weeping, unable to help him. I didn't argue when Lenny told the oncologist that he was declining the remaining two rounds of treatment.

Once again, we began to question why chemotherapy and radiation were the only conventional methods we had for destroying NHL. If cancer is essentially cells that are irregularly duplicating, wreaking havoc on the body due to a faulty immune system, certainly it would make more sense to find the root cause of the faulty immune system and fix it. Otherwise, the only alternative is to use drugs that will not only kill cancer cells, but could potentially wipe out the only healthy cells left in the body. This option only really leaves the patient with the hope that the cancer cells will die more quickly, leaving their body with enough strength to rebuild.

I knew I wasn't as educated as the doctors who were treating and caring for Lenny, but none of their treatments made any sense, and I knew Lenny and I weren't the only people asking these questions. The Reno clinic we had previously visited was using intravenous vitamin C treatments, an idea that originated in the 1970s with scientist, Linus Pauling, and Scottish physician, Ewan Cameron. While we hadn't pursued that particular treatment, it exists because Pauling and Cameron set up clinical studies observing the use of vitamin C to treat terminal cancer patients. According to their findings, vitamin C administered intravenously increased the patients' average survival time by four times that of patients who weren't given the same treatment.[10] While their findings were rejected by conventional medicine, Pauling was also credited with popularizing vitamin C as a supplement to help support the immune system against the common cold, a practice the majority of households use to this day, including my own.

Pauling and Cameron weren't the only ones to pursue alternative methods to treating cancer, and while we had a lot to learn and discover, I knew we weren't crazy for questioning the conventional treatments, even in the midst of using them as a last resort. Healing Lenny's immune system seemed like the best way forward, and so I did my best to encourage him to take supplements, eat a healthy diet, and sit in his sauna to help eradicate the residual chemotherapy drugs from his body. Eventually we received word that Lenny was officially in remission. The word tasted sweet in my mouth, and yet it was also almost too good to be true.

We celebrated Lenny'svictory, grateful that conventional treatment won this battle, and hoping that was also the end of the war. But remission is approached with a sense of caution, knowing that scans would be scheduled and blood work done in the months and years to come. There would always be a question in the back of our minds, asking whether or not cancer would return. If it did, I wondered what would happen to Lenny. Another round of radiation? Chemotherapy? More steroids?

Of course, in the moment, these thoughts get pushed around and then eventually pushed aside. Lenny was in remission, and maybe we didn't need to worry about anything beyond that. We shrunk the lymph nodes naturally, and we destroyed the

---

[10]   https://www.ncbi.nlm.nih.gov/pmc/articles/PMC431183/

spinal mass with chemicals. And maybe that would be the end of our story.

But it wasn't. When the cancer reappeared four years later, we knew we had to change direction again. The oncologist recommended a low dose of chemotherapy, Lenny declined. He realized that even seven years later the options were still the same: chemotherapy, radiation, steroids. Why had nothing changed?

The National Cancer Institute receives its four to five billion dollar budget—depending on the year— from the United States Congress, where certain amounts are allocated to different types of cancers or cancer prevention and control. Of those billions, currently $122 million is allocated to the research of Non-Hodgkins Lymphoma.[11] While it is difficult to understand where and how that money is used specifically, the general consensus is that research is pursuing new types of chemotherapy drugs, stem cell transplant methods, more targeted treatments, and immunotherapy. The reality at the time was that the only new option was simply a different type of chemotherapy. Same process, different chemical.

While millions may be spent on researching these new drugs and new methods, the patients turn around and pour thousands into purchasing those drugs. Chemotherapy costs differ depending on the type of cancer and the length of treatments, but the cost of any and all cancer treatments is continuously increasing. The more drugs that become available, the more expensive and less accessible they are.

Even in 2008, seven years after Lenny was diagnosed, we couldn't seem to shake the feeling that it was somehow all a ploy.

---

[11]   https://www.cancer.gov/about-nci/budget#current-year

We would pay thousands for treatment to then turn around a few years later and pay thousands more.

As we had done previously, we didn't completely abandon conventional medicine—it came through for us when we needed it most, and we had determined to seek healing from whatever method was available.

However, we redirected, turning our attention back to the realm of alternative medicine and trying to understand how to heal Lenny without causing further damage to his body. We certainly didn't have billions or even millions to spend on research, but we were determined, yet again, to find a solution.

CHAPTER SEVEN

Fight the Good Fight

There is only so much "they" can tell you to prepare you for the battle that is waged in the form of cancer treatments. Your hair is likely going to fall out. You may feel fatigued. Loss of appetite is common, just do your best to eat a healthy diet and drink a lot of fluid. Maybe they are just trying to ease you into the process, but I prefer a more realistic and authentic approach. "Here's what to expect," they should say, "the next six months will feel like hell. You will be exhausted. You will want to quit. The best thing you can do for yourself is find a reason to fight and then keep on fighting. Oh, and drink water, or you'll likely end up back in the hospital."

Traversing the path of cancer treatment is tough—physically, emotionally, and most certainly mentally. In fact, for Lenny, the mental fight proved to be where the battle was waged most aggressively. Treatments began with radiation, which didn't prove so challenging. He went for treatments twice a week for nearly a month, the doctors meticulously marking his body where the radiation would be focused. Gradually, the treatment melted the tumor off of his spine. The side effects were bearable—mostly fatigue. Sleep and a lot of grace from his employer got Lenny through the first month without much fuss.

Although the tumor was virtually gone once the radiation treatments were done, the oncologist recommended chemotherapy to fully eradicate any cancer that may remain. After hearing stories of other people's chemo experiences, Lenny felt he had a pretty good handle on what to expect. Hearing and doing are two very different things, however, and what Lenny didn't expect was the emotional and physical battle caused by such a small bag of chemicals.

The chemo room is well recognized among patients on the oncology ward. Everyone knows where it is, what it looks like, what it is for—no one wants to ever use it. Lenny and I had walked past that room many times, always grateful that we didn't have to go in. When you finally do have to enter that room, nothing quite prepares you for what's inside. Lenny's first round of chemotherapy was a day of unknowns: what would it feel like, what would the side effects be, how would his body respond? I went with him as moral support, although I could never really tell how much support I was really providing him. What did I know? How could I support him and protect him from this disease ravaging his body? I didn't have answers, and so I did what I could and stayed by his side.

I remember the look on Lenny's face when the nurses came into the room carrying a bag of chemo. He was on edge as they set the IV, and then he watched in apprehension as the purple fluid slowly drained into his body. We talked a little, while the fluid drained. The air in the room was heavy with anxiety and the weightiness of grief. Other chairs in the room held occupants of different ages, ethnicities and race. Another reminder that cancer doesn't discriminate.

Thanks to a pile of books and a portable DVD player that Lenny's work gifted him, we made it through the first round of chemotherapy and left the gloom of the room behind us as quickly as we could. And then we waited. It didn't take long for Lenny's body to respond to the chemicals coursing through him. He hit the bed and didn't emerge for several days, trying to survive what became known as the "hurricane effect," or what he later told me was the worst hangover imaginable, times ten.

We approached round two a little less innocently than we had round one. The purple chemical was no longer something to be apprehensive about; it was something to loathe. Lenny looked around the room again, contemplating the other patients when he realized that he was by far the youngest person there. "What the hell am I doing here?" he thought. We read, watched movies, chatted with the people next to us—when anyone felt like socializing—and let the purple chemicals slowly drip into Lenny's body. When the day was done, we returned home and waited for the storm to hit.

Chemotherapy, radiation, and the multitude of other cancer treatments are, as many have discovered, some of the most challenging treatments to endure. Chemotherapy leaves its victim exhausted, sore, and in some cases nauseated and weak. The more nerve-wracking side effects of treatment are much more harrowing: lung, kidney, heart or liver damage, not to mention irreversible damage to the reproductive system.[12] In most cases, your hair falls out. You don't feel like eating or hydrating or living.

Finding help, or at least finding someone to talk to about your cancer journey isn't difficult. Many facilities have someone available for counseling and encouragement. Lenny was assigned a social worker, a family counselor that was available to meet whenever needed, particularly throughout the treatments. We never met with her. Lenny didn't want to talk about how he was feeling and as much as I did, I wasn't really sure how to. We had no idea what we were up against.

As treatments continued, so did the array of mental and emotional challenges for which we were both utterly unprepared. You begin to grow accustomed to the faces and people sitting in the treatment room. Sometimes patients were there alone, and in an attempt to provide some semblance of comfort, I would make my way around the room, getting to know people who were willing to be known. One girl in particular appeared in the room one day; she was alone and she was young, much younger than Lenny. Our hearts went out to her. Again the questions surfaced—*why her, why any of them, God, why?* There was a woman there who Lenny recognized. She often staged and decorated the houses Lenny's company built. She was there one day, and by the next treatment she was gone. Suddenly it was no longer a question of why any of us were in that room, but who would last. Who would win and who would lose?

For Lenny, the world began to look a little different after that. He realized that we really can't take anything for granted.

---

[12]   https://www.cancer.net/navigating-cancer-care/how-cancer- treated/chemotherapy/side-effects-chemotherapy

You can be here one day and gone the next. We say those words, but when you face the reality of their meaning, something shifts in your very soul.

Jordan, our youngest, was just a baby, practically a newborn. Lenny began to wonder what Jordan's life would look like—his childhood filled with the battle that was raging around him, and the possibility of not having a father around to walk him through the days ahead.

Here is what else "they" don't always tell you about cancer: depression in chronic and terminal patients is very real and very prevalent. It can be difficult to translate symptoms experienced by cancer patients into the correct categories—depression and chemotherapy can both cause fatigue, loss of appetite, and loss of motivation. As far as the medical community can distinguish the symptoms, one thing is clear: depression and anxiety don't help the body in fighting cancer. In fact, one study revealed that "minor or major depression increases mortality rates by up to 39% and that patients displaying even few depressive symptoms may be at 25% increased risk of mortality."[13]

While these findings can be confirmed by multiple other sources, it still seems to be a minor part of the conversation.

[13]   https://www.ncbi.nlm.nih.gov/pmc/articles/ PMC4356432/#b5-ol-09-04-1509

How does someone keep a positive mindset after being told their life may be significantly shortened, that they are dying?

I remember the day that Dr. Speckhart, our alternative oncologist, told us that belief plays a huge role in fighting cancer. That isn't just belief in God or a higher power, but also a belief in one's purpose in the world and that their purpose will be achieved. A belief that cancer can be fought and defeated.

Finding that place of belief, however, is harder than it sounds, particularly in the midst of treatment. For Lenny, just getting through the day was difficult. The "hurricane effect" that the chemotherapy caused on his body was excruciating to watch, let alone experience. There was nothing I could do to make him more comfortable, and nothing he could do to subdue the pain and exhaustion. But somehow, one day turned into another and then another.

By the third treatment, Lenny's hair began to fall out. At first he thought it might stay put, he had already made it that far. As he was getting ready one morning, he put some gel in his hair when an entire chunk came loose in his hand. He began to pull more and more clumps of hair and they pulled free from his scalp with little effort. Finally, in resignation, he shaved his head. He began to understand why people give up on chemotherapy treatment—particularly patients who are already further on in life. Every three weeks, just as your body is starting to feel normal again, you put yourself through the horror of treatment. Sometimes, it feels like you would rather die than put yourself through that.

Lenny didn't want to die, however, and so instead he thought about Jordan. He thought about all of our kids and the childhoods they would have because of this. And he began to realize how desperately he wanted to defeat this disease. It had stolen enough, he determined, and it would not steal anything more. Anger began to fuel him. "My kids aren't going to know me," he thought, "and that's bullshit." His motto was simple: "'F' Cancer." It would not win.

He was on a mission. It was simple, really, what he made himself do. Even in the midst of chemotherapy, he would try to workout, staying as healthy as possible. Of course, that wasn't always possible given the "hurricane" days. But he kept going. On good days, he would do his rounds at work, despite the fact that they gave him an extraordinary amount of grace and insisted he rest. He liked the normalcy of a routine, and so he worked anyway. He couldn't put in a full day, just a few hours at a time, but it was enough to get him out of bed. It provided purpose.

Every day Lenny would find his reason to fight: our kids, our future, me.

Whatever or whomever he could hold onto, he would. When it seemed there wasn't much to hold onto, he would remember something a friend had said, some word of wisdom or question about life. Pondering it would make the day go by. When all else failed, he turned to rock and roll. "Fight the Good Fight" by the band Triumph became his anthem. He was facing his own fight, one day at a time, and he was determined to come out victorious.

Again, medical research shows us that over 70% of oncologists and 85% of patients believe that mood and mental well being impacts the patient's ability to fight cancer.[14] In fact, one theory suggests that authenticity, autonomy and acceptance play a role in a patient's ability to outlive their prognosis.[15] Ultimately, the hypothesis is that patients who know what is important in life, who feel they have the freedom to organize their lives around what matters most, and who have a greater sense of self-esteem, peace, and emotional connection with others are more likely to experience a slower progression of cancer and even help their bodies work to heal. Dr. Speckhart was correct, a lot of the journey toward healing has to do with what you believe.

In this way, Lenny methodically checked off each day, one at a time, until nearly eight months of treatments were completed and he was rewarded with remission. Lenny's drive was inspiring—he really did fight the good fight. He didn't fight perfectly—there were moments when seeking help would have been beneficial—but he did fight purposefully. The battle was won, but throughout his process, he continually asked God why he was going through this. What was the point? What was he supposed to learn? While these questions still remain, an answer came in the form of a friend.

---

[14]   https://www.ncbi.nlm.nih.gov/pmc/articles/PMC4356432/#b7- ol-09-04-1509

[15]   https://www.ncbi.nlm.nih.gov/pubmed/15312263

A few years later, a close friend of ours was diagnosed with a horrible case of leukemia. She was told that her best options were a high powered chemotherapy followed by a bone marrow transplant. Lenny recommended different alternative options rather than the transplant, but knowing that the option was hers, he also advised her on how to fight. "There will be days when you'll just want to die," he told her. "When you feel that way, you have to just hold on. Don't focus on that, because the next day is going to be a little bit better. Focus on getting to the next day." Six months after that, Lenny heard from our friend. She told him that his words got her through the treatment and helped her focus on beating the cancer. He had shown her how to fight.

Remission is a beautiful reward, but it is not easily won.

After the emotional shock of being diagnosed with a terminal disease, rediscovering a positive outlook on life can be difficult. Add to that the physical exhaustion of chemotherapy or any cancer treatment drug, and the emotional and mental strain on a cancer patient is profound. Despite the difficulty of the battle, however, depression doesn't have to be the reality for cancer patients, even if the prognosis leaves little room for hope. What are we here for? What are we living for? The same existential questions we all face as human beings are also in front of those fighting terminal diseases. The difference is a shortened timeline, a heightened sense that every day is a gift. Fight comes in different forms: anger, unwillingness to leave family behind, a drive to live out a purposeful existence.

Whatever it is that keeps us going, we are in it together—we need each other and we need purpose.

If authenticity, hope, and belief really do help our bodies combat disease, then I can only pray that we are all graced with an ability to fight the good fight. No matter what we are facing.

CHAPTER EIGHT

We're Still Standing...
We Can Beat Depression

When Lenny was told he was in remission, the sense of relief we felt was tangible, and we chose to let it dwell in and around us, for a moment, at least. The battle we had been waging for nearly four years was finally over and we were ready to put it behind us and begin again. Lenny and I both live in perpetual forward motion and we failed to see the moment as an opportunity for rest and recovery and instead interpreted it as our permission to begin our life together, without cancer.

Just as a weak immune system struggles to fight off disease, however, so too does a weakened emotional state struggle to fight off the residual strain of a long-fought battle. Lenny had won his immediate battle, and I was incredibly proud of him—not to mention relieved that he was still with us. Relief only lasts a moment or two, though, and then comes the train, and life, and suddenly we're swept away in its motion, all while still feeling broken inside.

Throughout his treatment, Lenny was laser focused, and there were days I couldn't access him—he was on his mission and I was the bystander cheering him on, although I desperately wanted to help him fight. He was on his mission and I was on my own; raising the kids, taking care of a baby, working and paying bills. Everyone copes differently, and I got through the long days and even longer nights by cuddling up with a bottle of chardonnay. Sometimes I would pray and other times I would yell at God, not sure if He was even listening. Worship brought me peace, at times, but all I could be sure of was the fact that if all else failed, two or three glasses of wine would be enough to help me sleep.

Depression isn't simply an issue among cancer patients or those dealing with a terminal or chronic illness. In fact, according to the World Health Organization, over 300 million people throughout the world struggle with depression on a daily basis.[16] A multitude of factors contribute to what the World Health Organization has designated a mental disorder: genetics, physical health, psychological health and even personality all contribute to both depression and anxiety, disorders that are very closely linked. Not only is depression increasing as a disorder, it is a contributing factor to ill health worldwide. Clearly, we have another war on our hands that goes beyond the one we are waging against cancer. And yet, they also go hand- in-hand.

---

[16]   http://www.who.int/news-room/fact-sheets/detail/depression

Caregivers and family members of those fighting long-term disease are also, equally at risk of dealing with anxiety, depression, and overall lower-quality of life. Your loved one is looking death square in the face, and therefore, so are you. How do we deal with the overwhelming sense of grief that comes as an unwelcome companion to fighting disease? How do you help someone face death and fight it?

What does it look like to live, make decisions, or plan a future with someone who might not be part of it?

These aren't the only questions we ask ourselves, and they certainly aren't always questions we consciously carry with us. These are the dilemmas, the existential crisis that our brains and hearts are dealing with all while we're sitting quietly next to our loved one in the chemo room. Sometimes in the midst of this crisis we even look happy. Because we have to. How else are we supposed to survive?

Our answer to these questions was simply to live. Sometimes that meant taking vacations we couldn't afford, and other times it meant avoiding the pain that was always just below the surface of our daily lives. On the simplest of days, living meant being together as a family, remembering that we were still here. When remission was declared, we celebrated and we took our family on a much needed trip away from the life we had been trying to survive. Lenny had just finished his last session of treatment and still looked like he was living in the hurricane, but we joined our friends at their beach house and we did the only thing we knew to do: spend time with our family, laugh, drink, celebrate, and enjoy the moment. Our photos of that trip juxtapose the craziness of our lives in that moment: we're laughing and smiling and Lenny's pale face and bald head are covered in white, chalky sunscreen. We still laugh at those photos. It was the first moment we remembered to have fun together.

Somewhere along the journey, Lenny and I began to joke with one another about our resilience. "Well, we're still here," we would say. If something broke down, there was a bill to pay, or Lenny would emerge from the bedroom after a particularly bad day. "I'm still here, aren't I?" he would joke. We would laugh and realize, yes, we are still here.

Depression can be hereditary. On my mother's side of the family there is mental illness as far back as you can go. The highs and lows that we faced over the first four years of our lives together would have been enough to cause even the healthiest person to struggle. Unfortunately, I was not the healthiest at that point in my life, and my predisposition to depression proved to be an obstacle I wouldn't be able to avoid. While Lenny was celebrating the high of winning his battle, I was about to be plunged into my lowest low.

I found that throwing myself into work, working out and cutting back on the chardonnay and caffeine helped with the ever present cloud around my mind. Busyness became my safeguard and a more considerate companion than a bottle of wine. I kept busy, Lenny returned to work, and we forged ahead.

At the time, we were living happily in the house we had built together, what we imagined to be our dream home. When a letter arrived from the city, all of that changed. A project to widen our road meant the city would be purchasing thirty-three feet of our front yard. This didn't just mean less front lawn for our family, it also meant that the road would be hosting more traffic and our little haven would no longer be a haven.

On a whim, Lenny and I began looking at houses out toward the country, away from the growing city. I had just listed a house out in Pungo, a suburb of Virginia Beach, and so Lenny joined me as I went to view the comps in the area. We stopped to look at a fixer upper with a gorgeous view when Lenny peeked over the bushes at the neighboring property. "Wow, babe!" he said excitedly. "Look at their setup." I looked over at a gorgeous florida-style ranch house with a deck and pool, overlooking about four acres of pristine landscaping. The property backed up to the canal and had four docks, a boat ramp and a huge boathouse.

I laughed at the sight of it. "It's not even for sale," I said, "and if it were, we couldn't afford it." Something about the property wouldn't leave Lenny, however, and so when we got home he asked me to pull up all of the listed properties in Pungo. I looked in disbelief as that ranch house appeared on the list. It had been posted just two days prior with a note, "There is no 'For Sale' sign and agent must be present by appointment only." Within minutes we were in the car headed back out to the property. We stood in the neighbor's yard and gazed through the bushes at the seemingly unattainable home. "Call your loan guy," Lenny said. "I'll sell the beach house."

That next weekend we had an appointment scheduled with the seller's realtor and we were headed back out to the country to view the property up close and on the inside. I had made up my mind that I wouldn't like it due to the long drive, the upkeep and, of course, the price. I told Lenny if it didn't have a big, open kitchen that it was a no- go for me. As soon as we walked in the house, however, we were blown away. The ceilings were vaulted in most every room, there was a place for everything imaginable and the kitchen was over 800 square feet of endless cabinets and countertops. Of course, it was completely open to the rest of the home. The agent, sitting at the bar in the kitchen looked at us and said in her country accent, "Is this kitchen big enough for you?"

Lenny asked me if he could talk to his realtor—me— before we signed on the bottom line. He asked me if I thought it was a wise investment. I explained to him that I had a knot in the pit of my stomach that wouldn't go away even when I prayed, and he said, "No that's my wife talking, I want my realtor's advice." I knew there was no backing down based on Lenny's body language and his facial expression and the fact that the property was more than we ever imagined we could own. I knew that owning the property was contingent on a few different factors: If we sold both of our homes and put additional money down, and if Lenny and I kept working at our current pace and salaries, we would be able to afford the monthly payment.

So I became Lenny's realtor in that moment. "Real estate is like any other investment," I said. "It goes up and down depending on the economy and because we are looking at a long term plan, we will probably be okay." That was in 2005.

What we didn't know at the time was that in less than three years, no one who owned real estate would be okay.

Prior to finalizing the contract, I had tried a litany of excuses for why we didn't deserve or couldn't afford the house. Or why it simply shouldn't be ours. My final excuse was a serious fear of snakes, and the property backed up to a canal that was most certainly home to a number of slithering creatures. I told Lenny that I wanted to go up the canal and walk the property again to see if I saw any snakes before we signed off on the final paperwork. He said I was crazy: there were definitely going to be snakes.

The seller assured us that she had only seen three to four snakes in the eight years she had owned the property, and that if you made noise when you go outside they would leave. I still needed to check it out for myself. After a long boat ride up several canals, we finally reached the backside of the property. I hadn't seen one snake. The boat captain— my first husband— said it was a sign from God; we should have seen tons of snakes. He agreed with Lenny that we should go forward with the purchase.

We signed a contract contingent upon selling our two homes and the seller accepted our terms and even gave us an additional six months leeway to sell our houses. We gave a ten thousand dollar non-refundable deposit and within six months, the Pungo property was ours. It was surreal, like living at a resort. After a day of showing houses, I would pull into our driveway and wonder how on earth our lives brought us to this place—this house and lifestyle.

The kids reaction to our new home was almost worth the worry that I was carrying around with me. They were thrilled to have a pool, a dock, a canal, and so much space to call their own. We loved to entertain, and the house was an entertainer's dream. We hosted friends whenever possible and had over two hundred guests in our backyard for Lenny's 40th birthday.

While life may never be perfect, there are moments that certainly give you a glimpse of perfection.

We were grateful for those moments.

Everything was good, on paper, at least. Lenny was well, our family was together, our house was beautiful. And then my brother passed away. Every un-touched emotion that had been simmering below the surface suddenly had no cap, no way of staying bottled up. I struggled off and on with depression since I was nineteen years old—the highs and the lows were not unfamiliar to me. Losing my brother, however, proved to be the catalyst that brought me to my lowest low.

Depression, despite the growing research and treatment, still very much has a stigma attached to it. What is it, really? A mental problem, an issue with your DNA, a physical problem, or a weakness? Are we over-diagnosing it in order to prescribe pills, or under-treating it because of the stigma? Today, in high-income nations nearly 50% of people diagnosed with depression aren't being treated, a number which dramatically increases in lower-income countries.[17]

Because we don't understand depression, it tends to be swept aside, avoided and ostracized.

"Just pull yourself together," we tell ourselves, "snap out of it." If only it were truly that simple.

My brother, who had been abusing alcohol for many years, was found dead in his home. Apparently he had added prescription pills into the mix of his already addictive lifestyle and the combination proved deadly. He was only forty one. The shock of his death was almost more than I could handle. I did my best to help my mother stay afloat in the midst of planning his funeral and all the preparations that go along with losing someone. Neither of us could sleep and we barely ate. I lost 11 pounds in a week and was struggling to cope. I knew my brother battled with addiction, but a new layer of guilt covered the grief—how did I not know his addiction was so bad?

Apart from the depression that runs on one side of my family, alcoholism has run rampant on my dad's side of the family going back seven or eight generations and to my knowledge has taken the lives of my grandfather, uncle, my brother and eventually my dad. They say that time heals all wounds, but even as I write these words the emotion of losing

---

[17]   http://www.who.int/en/news-room/detail/30-03-2017-- depression-let-s-talk-says-who-as-depression-tops-list-of-causes-of-ill-health

my brother is hard to control. I don't remember him as an alcoholic—that was his struggle but not his identity. When I think of him now, I remember his gift of cooking, his dry sense of humor, his crooked grin and his mannerisms that always made me laugh regardless of what kind of mood I was in. He was intelligent and miserable all at the same time, and in the end, the misery won.

Some organizations describe depression as a deep sadness. Others say it is a loss of motivation or enjoyment in everyday activities. Most agree that this sadness or loss of enjoyment, when occurring for a period of more than fourteen days, is in fact depression and not simply an emotional response to a circumstance or event. For me, depression went hand-in-hand with anger. Whether I was carrying around this anger my entire life, or not, it became my overwhelming and constant companion. During good periods—the highs—I could repress the anger, and pretend it didn't exist. That was not easily accomplished during the lows.

After my brother's death, the anger that spilled out from my life was almost incomprehensible. I hated the circumstances of our lives—the cancer, the fighting to survive, and the constant worry. I was angry with people for not supporting us except when things were outwardly difficult. I couldn't fathom why life was so horrible, why everyone was so horrible, and why God would let it all happen. I was really angry with God, but not as angry as I was with myself.

Self-destructive behavior, particularly suicide, is a common byproduct of depression. Not only are you swept into the black hole that is your mind, but because it seems that there is no escape, you find other ways to release yourself from the prison of hopelessness. Nearly every forty seconds someone commits suicide, and for every person that succeeds, an estimated 20 to 25 other people have attempted to take their own lives.[18]

It never occurred to me that I was truly at the worse stage of depression until the day I was taken away from my home in an ambulance, my children watching from the window. What started as thinning hair and rapid weight loss quickly turned into a cycle of getting through my days with no energy and outbursts of anger over the smallest things. I saw a doctor who prescribed several strong antidepressants, but those only heightened the already suicidal thoughts ravaging my brain. In my anger, I pushed everyone away and refused to be helped. If I couldn't love myself, how could anyone really love me?

The most trying moments of my depressive state brought about a three-month separation in which Lenny fought hard to keep me by his side. He wouldn't give up, and I couldn't understand why. Depression was not just a black emptiness, it was a state in which I made some of the worst decisions of my life. I hurt the people I love the most, and in doing so, added layer upon layer of guilt to my already unmanageable pile of anger, self-pity and grief.

I don't know that any one moment can be traced as the moment that brought me back to myself.

---

[18] http://www.who.int/mental_health/prevention/suicide/
suicideprevent/en/

If anything, grace was ultimately what saved me.

God's grace to slowly help me emerge from the cloud and a darkness that overwhelms. Lenny's grace in forgiving me and welcoming me home. And perhaps it was grace that also taught me to forgive myself for escaping down what felt like a never-ending path of destruction.

In the same way that Lenny learned how to fight through his treatments in order to defeat cancer, I learned that I also had to fight, but in my own way. I needed to learn how to accept help. Apart from the elements of depression that were hereditary or physical—I found out later I had entered early menopause—the act of being a caregiver had added an entirely new level of pressure to my life, and I hadn't sought any support. I remember going to work one day and a colleague asking me how I was holding up. It was a simple question, really. I burst into tears, however, as I realized I wasn't holding up. I was falling apart.

I am sure there are statistics about depression among cancer caregivers—the American Cancer Society has multiple pages of content about caregiving and advice for families dealing with cancer. There is even an entire website called "Help for Cancer Caregivers." Almost all the resources available will recommend getting help, talking to someone, sharing the load. In order to share the load, however, you have to be willing to ask for help.

One thing I have learned about myself is that I won't seek help until my face has hit the pavement. Throughout those first days and years of Lenny's fight with cancer, I constantly felt alone. Through no fault of their own, people would ask how Lenny was, how he was holding up, if there was anything they could do to help. I don't remember being asked how I was doing. At least not often. The more familiar question was, "How can I help?" I didn't know how anyone could help and I didn't know how to task people with jobs. How do you ask for help when you aren't technically the one suffering?

The worry that our family carried was another added pressure I hadn't expected. Conversations with relatives revolved around Lenny, what were we doing to help him? What diet was he on? Had we heard of such-and-such treatment? Everyone meant well and shared their opinions and thoughts with the utmost love. Had I been able to ask for help, or understand that I was drowning in the midst of everything, I know they would have rallied around me.

Sometimes, the littlest acts were the most profound.

Being asked how I was holding up was one of those moments. After that, I made a determination that if a friend was ill I would always ask the spouse or caregiver how they are and what they are going through. Another moment was the day some friends unexpectedly called and told us not to worry about dinner because pizza was on the way. That was it, something as simple as a pizza let us know that we were not alone. Lenny and I decided that showing up for people has a profound impact.

If someone is in need, we do our best now to simply do something about it rather than wait to be asked for help.

Because the truth is, someone may never ask for the help they need.

In learning how to seek help from others, how to show up and how to recognize my own needs I finally chose counseling. Talking to a therapist helped me deal with the stress of caring for Lenny and the grief of losing my brother. I was finally able to process my depression as well, recognizing patterns in my life that could be avoided in the future. I had to learn that no matter how high or low I felt, not to ride that wave. This was not a simple process, and it was certainly not a short journey. For two years I struggled with the pit of depression I landed in when my brother died.

Lenny has always had such a steady, stable attitude toward life. When things go wrong, his first response is to try to find a solution. With him, there is always an answer. For me, when life is outside of my control, I fall apart— mostly because I have let the burdens and stressors pile up over time. Through his steadiness, Lenny has taught me how to stay calm in the midst of chaos.

Learning how to let go of control and fear, however, was something only God could teach me. The chip that I carried around on my shoulder was a byproduct of repressed anger and unforgiveness. But what was I holding onto and why? I have always been very goal oriented, but at the end of the day, you can accomplish all your goals and do everything right and life can change in an instant. Life did change in an instant, and I was still holding on to the hurt and disappointment of those circumstances. It came down to this one reality: this person I adore is fighting this disease, and I can't control it. When I finally realized that I never would be able to control it, I was able to start healing.

Depression is not to be taken lightly—it is not something easily tossed aside.

Learning to love those around us and seeking to understand their daily reality is the first step toward helping those who struggle with depression and anxiety.

Offer help to those who might be incapable of asking for any themselves. Grace saved me when I was at my weakest. The love of my family helped me heal. Finding gratitude in the midst of pain helped me focus. That grace and love and gratitude would not have been possible without faith in a God who brings healing to those who suffer. Depression is not a kind master, but there is always hope to grab hold of. Find gratitude for the small things— your job, your car, your home—and the large things, like family and friends. When all else fails, find gratitude in every breath you take and remind yourself, "I'm still here, aren't I?"

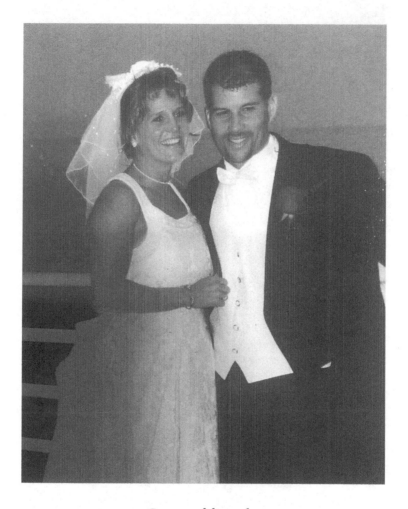

Our wedding day

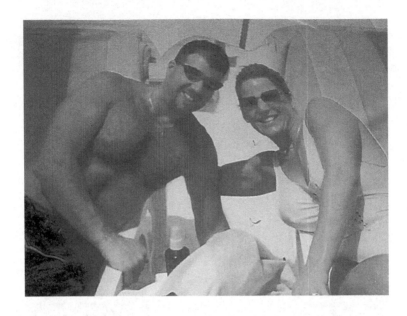

Our first trip together

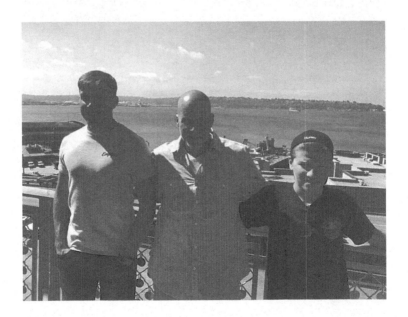

Seattle with Dylan

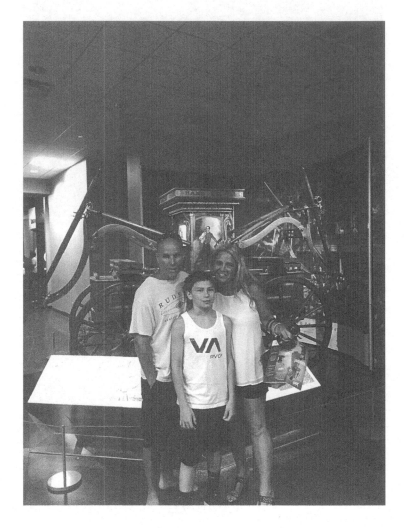

Our DC trip with Jordan

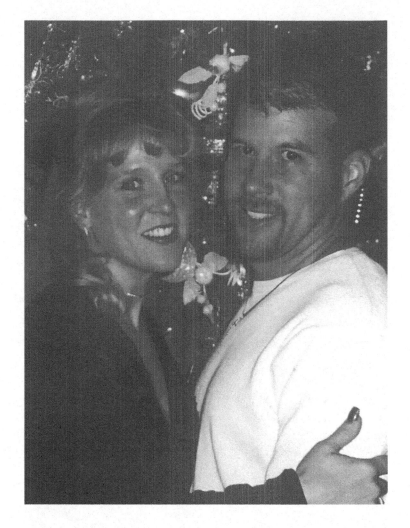

Christmas

A day to remember

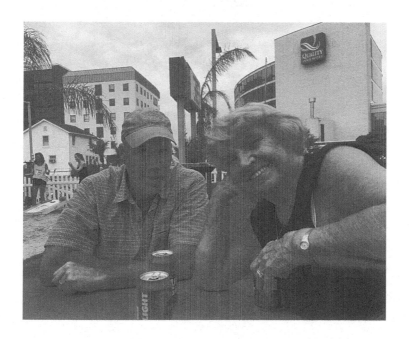

Lenny & Aunt Vicki

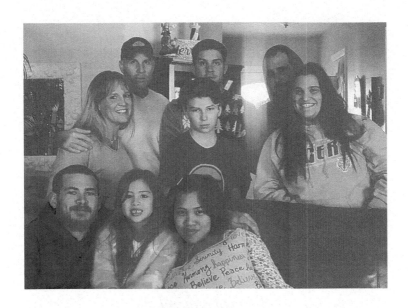

Family Christmas

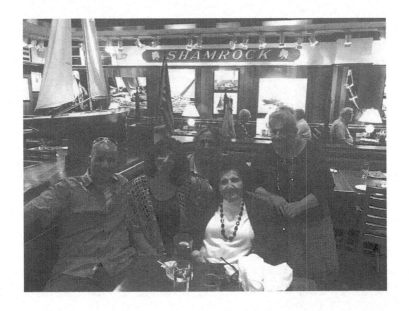

Lenny's mom, brother & sisters

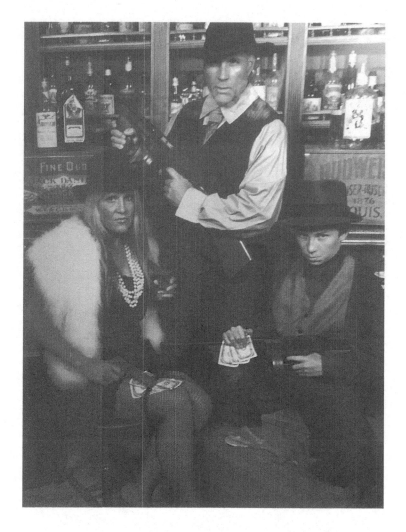

Family fun

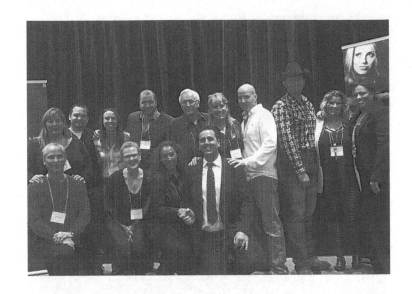

Our M Family

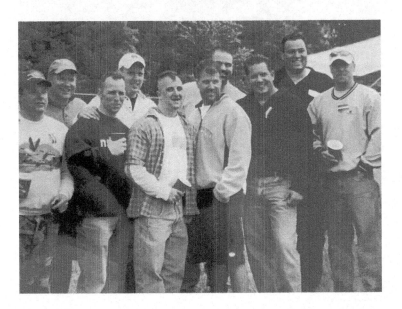

Lenny & the guys

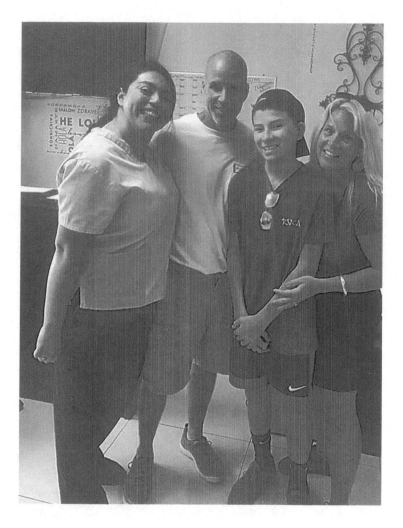

At the clinic in Tijuana

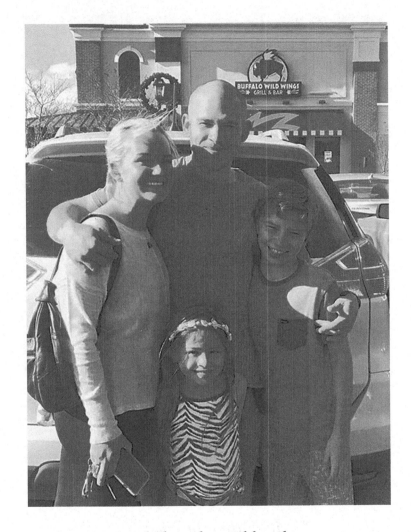

Our kids and granddaughter

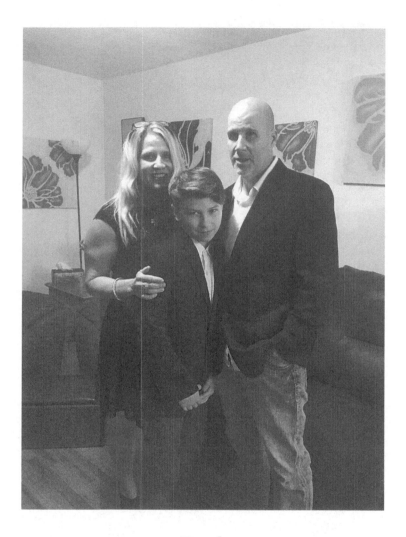

Family

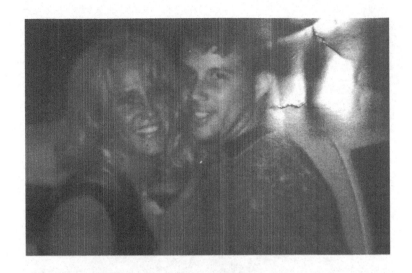

When we first met

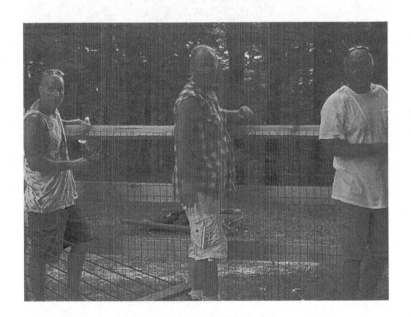

Lenny & his partners

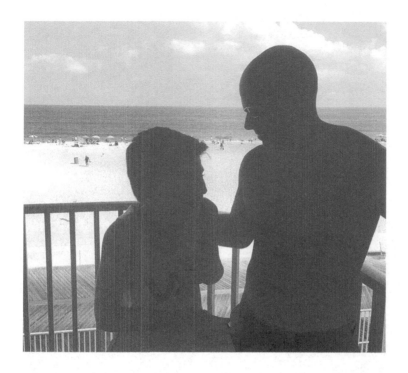

Ocean City

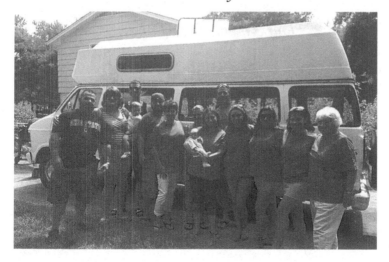

Team London

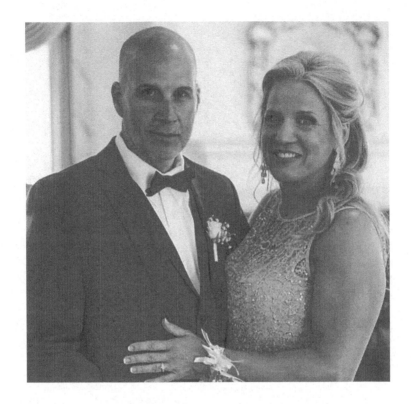

Our daughter's wedding day

CHAPTER NINE

Facing the Unknown

Remission is an interesting word. Like "malignant," or "benign," the sound of the word itself doesn't capture the essence of its true meaning. Strangely, remission can mean anything from the cancellation of debt to the forgiveness of sins, both of which are seemingly permanent resolutions to unfortunate situations. In the medical world, however, the word does not convey such permanence. When it comes to disease, the term merely communicates a respite, a temporary time of relief or a short delay. Some cancer patients do experience the respite from cancer for the rest of their lives, living in a perpetual state of remission. For those patients, we can't help but rejoice in their victory over the disease. Every individual triumph is a collective win for the community of people waging war on cancer. In those moments, remission is both beautiful and freeing.

On the other side of that word sits the unknown. Remission comes in different forms, from partial remission— the reduction of the amount of cancer in your body—to full remission or NED—No Evidence of Disease. Neither option, however, expresses what every cancer patient wishes to hear: that they are cured. Despite the sense of relief that comes with hearing a doctor say the word remission, it is difficult to ignore the lack of constancy in the prognosis. It means more tests and scans, setting up a regular watch- guard over the patient's body.

Lenny fell into the category of patients who experience remission as a temporary respite rather than an ongoing reality— for the time being, at least. He avoided his follow- up scans for several months until his sister and I were able to convince him to make an appointment. It was the end of 2008, seven years after his initial diagnosis with NHL. The scans showed enlarged mesenteric lymph nodes and Dr. Alberico recommended a round of low dose chemotherapy and Rituxan, a drug used to treat NHL and Rheumatoid Arthritis, among other diseases. The side effects include a warning that an allergic reaction to the infusion can result in death within 24 hours of the first treatment. Lenny denied both the chemotherapy and the Rituxan.

Remission may be a temporary reality, but it would not keep us from seeking different means of healing or wellness for Lenny. Around the same time, a close friend of ours called to invite me to a lecture in North Carolina featuring a doctor who had flown in from Tampa, FL. I agreed to drive south for the lecture, hoping that perhaps some of the products offered or discussed may at the very least, help Lenny's immune system. At the event, Dr. Brian introduced a new supplement product containing a key ingredient: resveratrol. Seven years had passed since that conversation at Johns Hopkins about the "resveratrol clinical trial study" that Lenny was too late to join. In that time, the few human clinical trials done to study the polyphenols effect on cancer and other diseases had been inconclusive. Lab studies, on the other hand, had revealed that the naturally occurring ingredient has incredible anti-inflammatory and antioxidant benefits, even proving to prevent tumor growth. Since the polyphenol naturally occurs in the skin of red grapes, it is often concluded that is the secret to the French Paradox: the very low rate of heart disease in a people group whose diet is high in saturated fats—and high in red wine.[19]

With lab trials giving the medical community plenty of hope for the uses of resveratrol, the slow pace of human clinical trials meant it was still not a viable treatment option offered in the oncological world. In the alternative and holistic world, however, it began to emerge as a popular supplement. At Dr. Brian's lecture, I grabbed hold of as many samples of the products as I could, in order to get Lenny started on them right away.

I learned that Dr. Brian, while initially studying chiropractic medicine, also studied nutrition and hormone therapy. I decided to have him order hormone panels for both Lenny and I. My hope was to find any issues that could be treated naturally. If Lenny's immune system was still struggling to combat the cancer, then it obviously needed some support. Much like the discovery of the Lyme disease, I felt like any information we could learn about Lenny's body would be helpful.

---

[19]   https://www.nature.com/articles/s41698-017-0038-6

What we discovered, however, is that while Lenny's hormones were balanced, mine were off the charts. Suddenly the struggle of the past two years made sense in terms of my physical and mental health. Too much estrogen, unbalanced testosterone and non-existent cortisol levels meant that even my antidepressants were rendered mostly ineffective on my imbalanced system. After just a few months of taking bioidentical hormones my hair began to thicken and my overall health and appearance improved. Complete balance would take a few years to accomplish, but the effect of just a few months of treatment were already enough to keep me going. I will always be grateful for Dr. Brian helping our family.

Lenny, in the meantime, continued taking various supplements and resveratrol. Choosing to decline the oncologists recommended treatments had not been a difficult decision. The memory of his previous treatment was fresh, as was the overall emotional weight of cancer. There is so much unknown about the disease, the treatments, the body's ability to fight and the potential natural elements available to aid it in that fight. Even during remission, the heaviness of the unknown is like a constant, weighty presence—for all of us.

The kids had grown up with cancer as a constant backdrop to their lives. While it didn't always impact them outwardly, and they weren't always cognisant of the battle going on, there was still the vague understanding that moments of hopelessness and struggle contradicted the usual drive and hope in the home. In middle school, my daughter struggled with the idea of death and dying. Counselling helped resolve what her young brain was trying to comprehend, but I realized how much this journey was impacting the lives of those around us.

Years later, the kids would tell us that what they sensed and noticed the most was how hard we fought and our unwillingness to give up.

Even in the face of the unknown, they noticed me sitting at my computer researching cancer treatments. They remember Lenny blasting 80's rock and roll every Saturday morning, his enthusiasm and humor saturating our home with a sense of normalcy and hope. Any moments of worry and fear were outweighed by Lenny's positive attitude and the belief that everything would be okay. I'm glad that we instilled hope and confidence in them, even in the midst of our worry and the unknown.

Lenny's dad had been living with us almost since the beginning, and while he proved an incredible champion and support for Lenny, he too carried the heaviness of everything he didn't and couldn't know about cancer. During the treatments, his worry increased. Was he watching his son die? Was the chemotherapy helping or killing? One day as Lenny lay on his bed, his dad came by the room to check on him. They made eye contact and Lenny said, "Dad, I got this. Don't worry about it."

Even in his weakest moment, Lenny did his best to take the edge of anxiety off of our household.

I suppose the unknown is as ever-present as the air we breathe. Everything we had walked through since the first diagnosis was unfamiliar—every day we were forced to make decisions in the face of everything we didn't know. We didn't know if resveratrol would help Lenny, or if denying chemotherapy was the right decision, but we moved forward anyway. We didn't know what the next years would hold, with our older children nearing the end of high school. We also didn't know that we were about to lose everything.

With the real estate market crashing in 2008 and 2009, my income went away overnight. I began working two part-time jobs to help pay the bills, and we made the decision to put the Pungo house on the market. It sat there for over a year. Since no one was looking to purchase million dollar homes in that economy, we instead tried to get a loan modification. Our request was denied eight times.

There were moments when I felt that perhaps this had been our own fault. Our excitement to live and not be held back by cancer, or anything else, had caused us to make spontaneous—and sometimes rash—financial decisions. The feeling I had in the pit of my stomach during the purchase of the Pungo home suddenly came flooding back to me. Whether it had been a premonition, discernment, or simply worry, I couldn't help but wonder what would have happened if we had heeded my gut instead of our confidence in the long-term investment.

Regardless of how we found ourselves in the situation, we couldn't control the real estate market, my income, or our mortgage company. So I did the only thing left to do: I called a local TV channel and sent them our hardship letter that had been denied eight times for the loan modification. The truth was, there was no reason we should have been denied as we qualified for the modification on several different counts. The local station agreed to run our story, but they also wanted to advocate for us. I laughed at that—I had been calling our mortgage company for the past year. Within hours of the TV station stepping in, however, we received a call from our mortgage company apologizing for the modification denial and stating they were in the process of approving our request.

The lower mortgage payments proved helpful, at least for awhile. We managed to stay in our home until the beginning of 2011 when Lenny was unexpectedly let go from his job. This change was about as shocking as the market crash. Lenny worked as a general superintendent for one of the largest builders in our area and, after 17 years, his income, benefits, and health insurance disappeared in a moment.

He came home that day with a look on his face that I will never forget. "I lost my job today," he said, almost matter-of-factly. He let me know that we would need to get him a new phone and a truck, since his current phone and truck were company-owned. "And we will need to go ahead and list the house as a short sale," he added, "because we won't be able to stay here."

There are a lot of things about that time that seemed difficult or overwhelming. We sold the house on a short sale for half of what we paid for it. Within weeks our retirement plan, Lenny's income, and our home were all gone.

However, despite the things that were lost, the biggest challenge for me was facing the unknown.

With every unexpected life event we experienced since our marriage, I thought perhaps by that point the unknown should feel familiar, like a friend who shows up unexpectedly at your door, but a friend nonetheless.

Facing the unknown, however, did not prove to be any easier with time. We had no backup plan, nowhere to live, and no money. My daughter, Diana, and Lenny's oldest son, Dylan, had just graduated from high school. Neither of them would be moving on with us as Diana was leaving for college and Dylan for the military. I suddenly regretted not knowing if they would have a home to come back to. We weren't just packing up our belongings, we were packing up the memories of a previous season. My oldest son, his wife and their daughter had also been living with us, and would be forced to find a place of their own. Lenny's dad was moving to Northern Virginia to an assisted living facility. We would suddenly go from a family of nine to a family of three. That felt like a far weightier loss than anything else.

With our life packed away in boxes, we drove Diana to college and said our bittersweet goodbyes. By that time we had decided to put our things in storage and live with my parents until a rental became available the following month. Our final day in Pungo we loaded the last of our things into a truck to move into storage. As I handed Lenny a dining room chair to add to the heap of boxes, he slowly turned and looked at me. "You know your life is F'd up," he said, "when you're putting all your shit in storage at age 40 and moving in with your parents." I couldn't agree more.

At some point or another, we all pray for humility, or at the very least seek to be a bit more humble than our egos would normally allow. It is my firm belief that one gains true humility when, in the midst of adulthood, one chooses to live with his or her parents. One month felt like an eternity. We lasted ten days with my mom. Her small condo proved to be claustrophobic after our full, but vast house. Our large lab, Sable, unwittingly added to the claustrophobia. We transitioned from my mom's small space to my dad's, which turned out far more crowded than our previous scenario. After three weeks of little sleep, Lenny, Jordan, the dog, and I all gratefully found ourselves in a temporary rental of our own.

When looking back on a timeline of your life, it sometimes seems to be tied up so nicely in this little package of events that happened at just the right moment and in just the right sequence. One horrible month can be summed up in a single paragraph. It is never truly that neat or simple or clean. Life is a mess and a mass of events that are thrown at you willy nilly while you do your best to swing and pray to God that you will hit the mark.

Life is a constant series of unknowns, sprinkled with seasons of "remission" here and there.

Daily life became a combination of work—Lenny started his own construction business—and taking care of one another. Lenny was still using natural supplements to try to reverse the effects of cancer in his body. I was also trying to help care for my dad who was dealing with multiple health problems including two strokes due to his lifelong alcohol addiction. After his second stroke, the doctor explained to my dad that if he didn't make drastic changes to his unhealthy lifestyle that the next stroke would end him. He was in the hospital and rehab for nearly two months, and I was convinced that I alone would make him change his habits. When he returned home, I instructed his caregivers that he was not to be given alcohol under any circumstances. Instead, my dad simply joined an online wine club and had the bottles delivered to his house. I was absolutely incensed watching my dad slowly drink himself to death while my husband fought so hard to stay alive.

In Northern Virginia, Lenny's dad had a bad fall which put him in the hospital and eventually a nursing home. His aging body was slowly declining, and it was not many months before he passed away. Daddy Jack, as we often called him, was thought to have had cancer toward the end, but his age and health meant treatment wasn't really viable. Instead, the family gathered around him and said our farewells, offering him as much comfort and connection as possible.

I'll never forget watching Jordan at the funeral. He showed hardly any emotion until the viewing when he looked at his grandpa in the casket. He began to weep and turned away with tears streaming down his face. Daddy Jack had lived with us since before Jordan's birth and was a constant in his life. Losing Jack made losing the house feel meaningless; it was replaceable, but he was gone from our daily lives. I believe we will see him again someday, when we all make our way to eternity, but the loss of his presence on earth will always be felt.

A few months after Daddy Jack's funeral, we experienced the unexpected loss of my dad. No one got to say a proper goodbye like we had with Lenny's dad. Instead, my dad was found one morning on his bathroom floor. He had died of a stroke. I had known this day would come eventually, but regardless of how prepared we are, loss and death bring grief and sadness. The day he passed, I drove over to his condo to make preparations for his body to be taken to the funeral home. I was waiting in the lounge with my cousin when the doorbell rang and I answered it, expecting to see the coroner. Instead, there stood a woman holding a box of wine in one hand and case of beer in the other. A strange sense of relief swept over me when I realized that my dad wouldn't have to fight his addiction any longer. His battle was finally over, and just like Daddy Jack, we would cross paths again one day when loss and disease are no longer ours to bear. Our fathers had received their remission—their eternal respite from life's journey.

Facing the unknown is still not familiar, or comfortable in any way. It is, however, necessary. When Lenny was diagnosed with cancer, we were overwhelmingly unfamiliar with the landscape we were about to traverse. I did my best to control what I could: the pursuit of healing, the financial health of our family. On the other end of depression, I had finally started to realize how little control I really have. When it came to losing our home, our livelihood, and our fathers, we were humbled to the point of letting go of all we thought life should and would be. They say life is a journey, but sometimes the journey isn't tangible forward motion. It is a meandering of the heart as it finds its way to understanding and peace with the unknown.

CHAPTER TEN

Healing at Any Cost

In 1873, Horatio G. Spafford penned the famous lyrics to the hymn "Ville du Havre," named for a ship that sunk in the Atlantic, taking with it the lives of his four daughters. As Spafford traveled from the United States to Europe to meet his wife, the only family member to have survived the wreck, he contemplated all that had happened to him over the span of just a few years: the death of his young son, the Great Chicago Fire that destroyed his real estate investments—and his fortune—and now the death of his remaining children. The words he wrote in response to his loss have been sung in churches around the world, crossing denominational lines and speaking directly to the truth of the human plight. Loss and sorrow are universally understood, and so is the desire to find peace in the midst of chaos. In the deepest moments of pain, Spafford wrote these words: "When peace, like a river, attendeth my way, when sorrows like sea billows roll;

whatever my lot, Thou hast taught me to say, it is well, it is well with my soul."

From our position, we had not encountered the level of loss that Spafford experienced: I still had my children and my husband, despite the other losses we had sustained.

The depth of pain we experience as humans, however, is real no matter the circumstances that caused it.

Devastation is not a competition—it is an invitation to discover peace. Spafford did more than write some beautiful lyrics, he demonstrated what it looks like to be well in soul—to find peace when loss surrounds you.

Over the next few years, we experienced a deep settling over our lives. My oldest son, Blake, and his family lived nearby, Dylan was stationed in Texas and was thriving in the military, and Diana blossomed in college. Jordan was making new friends and adjusting to a new school, and we even decided to adopt. Our new child was a white lab puppy that we lovingly named Simba. Peace and gratitude reigned supreme as we celebrated life every day. The words of the hymn rang true—it was well with our souls.

I found a rhythm of life that kept me grounded—satisfied, even. Every morning I would throw on my gym clothes, switch on some worship music and go for a walk or a run. Endorphins soothed my mind and the worship soothed my spirit. I had slowly begun to reduce my hormone intake, and had managed to work my way down to the lowest dose of Wellbutrin to keep the depression in check. My body was returning to normal.

Further healing came when a couple from my church generously sponsored my attendance of a three-day faith retreat. I attended Walk to Emmaus, an inter-denominational event for people to experience and grow in their understanding of faith in Christ. For me, it was three days of pure love and support, something I had been needing since the beginning. I finally understood how important it is for caregivers to ask for help, and how valuable it is when help is offered. I remember well-intentioned people showing up to talk about their uncle's, sister's neighbor who died of lymphoma, and how it would break me. But when people just brought food, and love, it was healing. Walk to Emmaus solidified the peace of mind that marked that season of our lives.

Every caregiver needs an opportunity to be loved on and supported in a way that speaks to their belief and well-being.

Mine couldn't have come at a better time.

After declining treatment at the end of 2008—taking resveratrol and natural supplements instead—Lenny's scans remained mostly clear for a number of years. That particular winter, however, Lenny's scans revealed devastating news. The cancer had not only spread, creating a 33 cm mass in his abdomen, but had morphed from Small Cleaved Cell to a more aggressive, Diffuse Large B-cell Lymphoma. Again, we found ourselves at the crossroads of conventional and alternative choices.

Because of the aggressive nature of the new cell type, time was of the essence, and other methods were available to Lenny that hadn't been with his previous diagnosis. The previous cell type was slow and steady, and incurable. Dr. Speckhart, our alternative doctor told us in the beginning that while it was not curable, it was maintainable. Through both conventional and natural treatments Lenny had, at that point, maintained for 12 years. But this was an entirely new beast.

Lenny's oncologist, Dr. Alberico, recommended radiation, chemotherapy, and a stem cell transplant, the end goal being an entirely new immune system and a body free of cancer. "Health at any cost," we reminded ourselves. So we took a deep breath and leapt. Lenny pulled out his old Triumph CD, found his fight, and plunged headlong into nearly a year of treatments.

Because of the location of the tumor in Lenny's abdomen, Dr Alberico took precautionary measures and had Lenny hospitalized each time he went in for chemotherapy. The tumor was near Lenny's intestines, and the oncologist was worried about tiny intestinal holes being created as the tumor was shrinking. With a surgeon nearby should that occur, Lenny began radiation and an aggressive series of the RICE chemotherapy cocktail.

One thing cancer patients come to learn is that chemotherapy is never one drug entering your bloodstream, but a series of drugs, through IV, injection and a litany of pills.

113

Every drug in the RICE cocktail has different side effects, so along with the chemotherapy comes anti-sickness drugs, antihistamines, G-CSF to help your body produce white blood cells, and Mesna—to prevent bleeding in the bladder that is a common side effect of ifosfamide, the "I" in RICE. The three-day rounds of treatment were far more intense than the original R-CHOP cocktail that Lenny endured years before. While the symptoms and side-effects were slightly different, the pattern of his life became a familiar rhythm: fight, sleep, repeat.

This time, we weren't as naive as we walked through the treatment process. Research still left us baffled about the extraordinary amount of side effects and possible issues caused by the four RICE drugs entering Lenny's body. Apart from the risk of infection, bleeding, bruising, and hair loss, the drug combo can also cause your tumor to break down so quickly that it releases uric acid into your system, sometimes more than your kidneys can handle. To prevent this, yet another drug is given to the patient. Drugs to prevent the negative effects of drugs. At times if felt like an endless cycle.

Thankfully, Lenny made it successfully through the next six months of radiation and chemotherapy. He did not endure any holes in his intestine, although we were grateful for Dr. Alberico's precaution. At the end of his treatment series, Lenny's stem cells were extracted for his upcoming transplant. They were housed at the Red Cross while Lenny received a two-month break to allow his body time to recover from the chemotherapy.

In September of 2014, we went to the hospital for Lenny's transplant. He would be there for 21 days. For the first time in many years, we had an incredible amount of hope that the chemotherapy and the stem cell transplant would work, bringing Lenny to the end of his fight with cancer. Lenny's stem cells were perfect after the chemo and radiation and they would hopefully help him build a brand new immune system. Dr. Alberico, too, had hope and encouraged us that this time we were going for the cure.

Having finally learned to ask for help, I called on our family to take care of Jordan and the dogs while I stayed with Lenny in the hospital. The first five days Lenny was put on a round of the strongest chemotherapy available. I watched as he struggled with the drugs coursing through his body, his eyes looked bloody and his mouth was "on fire." Nothing soothed his pain, no matter how many ice chips or cups of water I gave him. My heart ached for him and I silently prayed for grace and for the pain to leave Lenny's body.

When he had undergone enough treatments that his body could no longer rebuild its own cells, he was ready to receive the transplant. His blood counts were so low that he had to be isolated to prevent him from getting an infection. Despite his isolation, we invited our pastor in to pray for Lenny prior to the transplant.

We were nervous, but peace and hope prevailed as Lenny received what we prayed would be his last cancer treatment.

On October 7th, 2014 the transplant was completed and the hospital staff came in to Lenny's room to celebrate what they called his "new birthday." After almost 12 months of treatments, I sat watching Lenny cracking jokes with the staff and loving on his family. He was filled with hope and I was overcome with gratitude.

Hope, alone, felt like a victory.

As Lenny recovered, friends and family came by to celebrate with us. My two closest friends showed up a few days later with cake and balloons—to celebrate my birthday and Lenny's new one. It felt like the best birthday in years, surrounded by the people I love, holding the man I love, and having hope for life. In that moment, it was well with my soul.

Of course, the true test of how well our soul is prospering is in the times of strife and disappointment, not just the moments of joy. After Lenny's transplant, we waited for the follow-up scans. It felt like an eternity. We finally received the promising news: the majority of the tumor was gone and the standardized uptake value (SUV) was less than 5%. The doctor assured us that the 5% abnormality could simply be scar tissue, and so we scheduled the next round of scans.

We weren't sure how to categorize the scan results after the battering Lenny's body received in the last round of therapy. It was promising, but it also wasn't remission. Only time would tell us if the transplant had done its job completely, so in the meantime, Lenny was set on having a plan in place should the next scans show more cancer. We began researching cannabis oil, a topic that had come up in conversation (and online) over and over again. We sat at our computers and read testimonial after testimonial of former cancer patients who had killed the disease by ingesting the oil.

At first, I was taken aback at Lenny's adamant pursuit of finding a way to make some cannabis oil. He had never even smoked a cigarette, let alone taken any illicit drugs. He was, however, very open to taking this oil. Not being well versed in the use of even medical marijuana, we weren't sure where to find it or how to make the oil once we got our hands on the plant. The research kept leading us to something called Rick Simpson oil, so we found Rick Simpson's website and Facebook page. Both sources had tons of information about how to make the oil and details about plants to use. There were also several warnings to avoid fake oils, urging the public to find a reliable source of the plant and make the oil at home. I decided to email him Lenny's story and ask for advice. He answered by pointing me back to his website, telling me that if I can make a pot of coffee, I can make my husband's oil.

I began asking family members and friends if they knew anyone who might be able to help. No one seemed to have any answers or connections, and I felt like we had reached a dead-end. How was I supposed to infiltrate this world of which I knew nothing? A few weeks later, out of the blue, I received a call from a former colleague and friend. He was calling to ask how Lenny and I were doing and to let me know that his mom was also battling cancer. I told him about the transplant and scans, and our recent endeavor to find or make some cannabis oil. He immediately called his brother on the West Coast and asked him if he would be able to get access to the correct plant. He could, and within two weeks I was on a plane headed out west.

To say I participated in this lightly would be a lie. I prayed—and I prayed hard—about whether or not it was right to make this oil.

My love for Lenny overruled any fear or doubt I felt about marijuana.

With a group of "underground" supporters around me, I embarked on what lovingly became known as "Operation Lenny."

My hosts were delightfully helpful, taking me around to the stores to buy the ingredients and supplies for the oil. A friend of theirs even joined the operation, lending her know-how from working with several growers and medical marijuana shops. At the liquor store, our arms full of alcohol, a group of men asked us where the party was. "No party," my companions responded, "this is for Operation Lenny!"

We spent the next eight hours following the step-by- step instructions from Rick's website. He was right, if you can make a pot of coffee, you can make cannabis oil. By the following morning I had several syringes of oil—what I hoped would be Lenny's answer. Later that morning, my hosts took me to pick up my rental car and I was on my way back home.

I drove as far as I could each day before finding a hotel to stay in for the night. I would hit the road early the next morning, eager to get back to Lenny. Everything was going as planned until I was driving through Indiana and a K-9 trooper started following me. I'm almost certain my heart stopped beating. I called Lenny and asked him if the K-9 on his truck meant that he had a dog with him. He assured me it did, and I panicked. I'm not sure what I imagined would happen, but I was sure if he had a dog he would pick up the scent of the cannabis in the car.

The next 40 minutes seemed to be the longest of my life as this police officer stayed close on my tail. At one point, he got off the highway and I breathed a sigh of relief. As I approached the next toll booth, there he was again, this time in front of me. As I paid the toll, the lady taking my money looked at me suspiciously and scanned the inside of my car. I told myself that I was just being paranoid and quickly pulled away from the toll booth. Before I knew it, the officer was behind me again. That's when I began to pray. "Jesus, let him get a call," I prayed, "Let him be pulled away to something else more important!" I kept a close watch on him in my rearview mirror, when suddenly he pulled to the highway median, made a u-turn and drove off in the opposite direction.

I was on edge for the next 24 hours as I drove the final leg of the trip. I was convinced that K-9 officer had been following me, waiting for a reason to pull me over. As I drove into West Virginia, I called my daughter and she convinced me to make the slight detour to visit her. I pulled into her apartment complex the next morning and she ran down to greet me. As she opened the car door, her face contorted and she said, "Mom! That smell!" She ran back into her apartment and came back with a bottle of Febreze, spraying it all over the car and trunk. I laughed. Apparently I had become immune to the strong odor. But maybe the K-9 dog really could smell it on the highway? I guess we'll never know. Diana and I enjoyed catching up over breakfast, and when she went off to her classes, I got back on the road.

Lenny and Jordan welcomed me home as if I had been gone for months, and in some ways it felt like I had. Making and harboring cannabis oil had stretched me and also somehow rejuvenated me.

It felt like I had traversed a long and distant road to bring a possibility home to my husband.

Whether or not it worked, it was worth it. "It's for the love of Lenny," I told myself.

Lenny decided not to begin taking the oil until after his next scans, that way he could more easily monitor his progress. He had been right to pursue a back-up plan, and the oil arrived home just in time: his scans showed new cancer cell growth. He felt defeated and frustrated. The transplant was supposed to be his answer, his brand new immune system, his cancer-free body.

He denied any further conventional methods and instead began taking the cannabis oil. For the next four months, Lenny ingested the oil and diligently tried to get up to the recommended dose of one gram per day. As hard as he tried, he couldn't seem to ingest that much oil. Even half a gram made him high and we realized the strain of marijuana was just too high in THC for his body. He carried on anyway, taking as much as he could until his next scans.

We shared some of the oil with a few friends who were also battling cancer, one of whom had received so much chemotherapy that she experienced extreme bone pain. She had already been smoking cannabis to relieve the pain, and had refused any more chemotherapy, despite the two spots of cancer growth on her scans. A few months after adding the oil to her daily regimen, her scans came back cancer-free.

Unfortunately for Lenny, the cannabis oil did not have the same effect on his body. The scans showed that his tumor had doubled in size in a matter of months. We were crushed. Lenny declined the recommended treatment—40 rounds of radiation and chemotherapy. Nothing had changed, and we felt like nothing ever would. The answer from the medical world was always the same: chemotherapy and radiation. "How do we fight this, now?" I asked God. "How do we keep fighting a losing battle?" In the midst of my discouragement, I lost sight of hope and peace. My soul was not at all well, and for a time, I wondered if it would ever be well again.

Lenny told us that he was through mortgaging his body for conventional medicine. Seeing my reaction to his scans and worried that any added stress would put me over the edge, he instructed his family not to call me during that time. Instead, he asked them to help us research and find a solution other than chemotherapy or radiation. We would find a better way, he insisted. We had to.

The question that kept rolling around my mind was, what if it never totally goes away? What if the cancer is part of our lives, Lenny's life, forever? Can we live with that? I knew that we would always fight, of course we would fight. We would pursue healing because we love Lenny and because he's worth it. But in the midst of the fight, could we find peace and rest? Could we learn to be okay with ourselves?

In the Bible, there is a verse—a prayer, really—that perhaps Horatio Spafford used as inspiration for his hymn.

"Beloved, I pray that you may prosper in all things and be in health, just as your soul prospers" (3 John 2 NKJV).

That is what we needed, to prosper, be in health, and be prosperous in our souls. I started to ask different questions, ones not based on fear, but hope. What if, I wondered, Lenny never does another radical, poisonous thing to his body and lives for another 30 years?

And so I prayed. I prayed that we would prosper and be in good health. I prayed that we would find a natural option to heal Lenny's body, and I prayed that we would be okay—as a family, as husband and wife. I thanked God for how far we had come, and the victories that we had already won. I thanked Him for Lenny and his drive to find solutions. I prayed and Lenny searched—determined as ever in his pursuit. Together we found balance and peace again. And while I prayed, Lenny found the solution he had been searching for.

CHAPTER ELEVEN

Miracles Happen in Mexico

At times, I would wonder how it took us so long to come across things like the cannabis oil, or resveratrol. Why is it that there was so little support and information available? How is it that we would struggle to discover resources and options that had been available for years? But then I remember: when Lenny was first diagnosed, the internet wasn't part of our everyday lives. Facebook didn't exist, wifi receivers weren't magically built in to your computer (if we even knew what wifi was at the time), and chat rooms were seedy places where conversations took place with faceless, nameless strangers. Nowadays you can find countless cancer support groups on Facebook, cannabis information is all over the internet, and the American Cancer Society's website even has its own cancer survivors network and chat forum.

I came home from work one evening and Lenny was sitting on the couch with his iPad. He called me over, wanting to show me something. I joined him on the couch and he pulled up a video on YouTube and pushed play. Curious, I watched as a woman shared from her heart her story of how she had been diagnosed with NHL ten years earlier. She had opted for conventional treatment, but when she had a horrible reaction to chemotherapy, her doctor sent her home saying there was nothing more he could do.

She went on to share about how her husband, through much research, found a clinic in Mexico that offered several types of alternative treatments. Not knowing what else to do, they took a leap of faith and went to Mexico. She responded well to the treatments and went home after a few weeks completely healed. That was 11 years ago. She has been in remission ever since.

For the next several weeks, Lenny and I researched the clinic in Mexico, weighing the pros and cons and watching testimonials. Throughout our research, I kept thinking about the lady who was healed of NHL. If the clinic's methods worked for her, why not Lenny? We decided to go to Mexico, of course. We had come this far, hadn't we? Our friends and family seemed concerned for our safety when we announced what we would be doing. At times I even wondered if they thought we were a little bit crazy. And maybe we were.

Lenny always chuckles when we talk about our trip and says it was the longest six weeks of his life. For me it went by in a flash. It was an adventure and full of the unexpected. Despite all of our research, we really had no idea what we would encounter once we got there. We decided to leave Jordan at home in the care of friends and family. Within a few weeks of watching that first video on YouTube, we said our goodbyes and flew into San Diego. Our plan was to go back and forth between San Diego and Tijuana, feeling much more comfortable with the idea of staying at a hotel in California. There was a shuttle that would take us back and forth, and as far as we could tell, it was a great plan.

The first day the shuttle sat at the border crossing for over an hour. The driver informed us that some days it can take up to three hours to get over the border, so as soon as we got to the clinic, we set out altering our hotel arrangements. The clinic itself was in a very old, rundown three-story building in the heart of Tijuana. Lenny and I immediately felt at home and welcome in that space. The people greeted us with such warmth and we were surrounded with a sense of peace. As we approached the reception, I saw a little sign sitting on the desk: "Miracles Happen Here."

After consulting with the patient advocate at the clinic, we were given a list of nearby hotels. We found one just a mile down the road that offered discounts to clinic patients. I laugh to think about our plan to shuttle back and forth. A mile down the road, we had a pool, three restaurants and a higher rating than our hotel in California. We also felt safe, which was by far the most important aspect. The plan, according to all of our previous phone conversations with the clinic, was to be there for three weeks. We would follow the daily regimen and Lenny would received treatments. The days became very routine, for me as well as Lenny.

Monday through Saturday we would wake up around 7 am and walk over to the clinic for breakfast. The first hour of the day was spent eating and getting to know the other patients and their families.

For the first time, Lenny felt like he wasn't alone in the battle.

His hospital experience in the United States carried the distinct essence of fear, seclusion, and cautious optimism. In the Mexico clinic we were surrounded by warmth and curiosity, determination and faith, not just in God, but in humanity.

Lenny was the longest surviving patient at the clinic, and the other patients and guests wanted to know what he had done to survive the battle for what had now been nearly 16 incredible years. What did he eat? What supplements did he take? Did he do chemotherapy or radiation? How did he stay so positive? Something that I had known since the beginning, but couldn't quite put into words, solidified for me in Mexico. Back home, every time we tried something new, whether traditional or alternative, it was received with doubt and hesitancy. While we had embraced the fight and the willingness to try anything, the wider community—our society—only offered criticism and fear. Those trying to provide unconventional therapy were labeled as frauds. Doctors who wanted to offer their patients a holistic approach were looked down upon, and the entire system is ruled by pharmaceutical companies who, it would seem, care about their profit more than the overall health of the patient.

In this tiny clinic in Tijuana, we finally experienced a community of people who understood how to embrace the tension of pursuing life in the face of doubt.

For sixteen years we lived on a constant, unsteady rollercoaster of hope and defeat, belief and doubt, confidence and fear. Nothing was ever steady, except perhaps our love for one another, and God. Everything else was a whirlwind of choices, some based in fear and others based in faith. Suddenly, we were around people who understood the chaos of that journey. Our new group of friends valued the options, even the ones that looked ridiculous to the outside world.

The most beautiful aspect was the partnership of doctors and patients all working toward a common goal. Medical advancements lived alongside creative, out-of-the-box thinking and worked together for the greater good. I know that is the foundation of the medical community worldwide, it is, after all, the essence of the Hippocratic Oath—to consider the patient's entire wellbeing, avoid over-treatment, and seek to prevent disease, not just find a cure. However, our modern world is overrun with fear and strife and doubt. We take what the FDA approves at face value, and toss aside ideas that challenge our understanding of what is healthy or right.

In our pursuit to kill cancer cells, we've lost sight of what it means to make people well again.

Sitting at the breakfast table in Mexico, we were surrounded by many who were just beginning their fight against cancer, and to them, Lenny was a miracle. I was reminded that I've found him to be a miracle all along. Every time we tried something completely radical or even mainstream, it has impacted the cancer in Lenny's body. Even chemotherapy and radiation played their part in reducing cancer growth, at least for a time. From Dr. Speckhart's supplements and sauna treatments to resveratrol, changing his diet, and even just his determination to fight—all of it has resulted in Lenny's ongoing miracle.

For me, our time at the clinic was unlike any of Lenny's previous series of treatments. I felt closer to him than ever before, and I felt embraced by a new band of brothers and sisters who were also fighting for their spouse, parent, or child. It was a new kind of support system and one I will cherish forever. Lenny and I were able to offer encouragement to those who had also tried many different options and therapy methods. In fact, we all encouraged one another as living examples of what it looks like to stay in the fight.

Over the course of three weeks, Lenny did fourteen different therapies. Many of them were unfamiliar to us, different heat and light therapies, IVs of Vitamin C, Curcumin, and B17—or laetrile. One particular machine, called the Rife, was so effective that we decided to purchase one for our home. The machine uses electromagnetic frequencies believed to both identify and target the cancerous cells in the body. Like many of the alternative methods we have come across, there have been no large, controlled clinical studies done on the benefits of the Rife machine, so it remains a fringe treatment for cancer. Lenny felt an immediate effect from the machine, and uses his to this day.

The clinic also had Lenny take a low dose chemotherapy coupled with DPT to help the chemo cocktail specifically target the cancer cells and not his healthy ones. This method meant the side effects of chemo were very limited since the healthy cells weren't being destroyed by the chemicals. In between the therapies, Lenny would see his floor doctor and the main clinic doctor twice a week to go over scans and test results. His body responded quickly to the therapy.

During the first week, however, the clinic doctor—who Lenny affectionately referred to as the Godfather—encouraged Lenny to stay an extra three weeks. We were taken aback and a little disappointed, even hesitant. We spent some time processing this, talking to other patients, and questioning the doctor as to why the clinic didn't prepare patients in advance for this possibility. After our initial hesitancy, and several days of seeing Lenny's body respond to treatment, we decided to stay the extra three weeks.

Our days consisted of breakfast together as a group followed by five to six hours of therapy. After therapy we would have lunch together before heading back to our respective hotels. Part of the treatment process was spending time with Chef Raul, who showed us how to cook simple, healthy recipes that would be the most beneficial for our patients. Breakfast and lunch were provided at the clinic as part of our introduction to a healthier diet. Throughout the process, I kept thinking about the number of hospitals in the United States that offer sugar-riddled foods that lack any nutrients.

Children in cancer wards are brought pudding and jello, when their bodies are fighting to stay alive. I took my time with Raul seriously and endeavored to learn the recipes so that I could replicate them at home. In the beginning, I remembered telling Lenny that we needed to change his diet, and for the most part, we had. However, the abundance of information at the clinic changed my perspective even more and our diet radically changed.

During the five or so hours of therapy, family members would wait in a separate room since the treatment room was only large enough to accommodate the twenty or so patients receiving therapy. We would take turns visiting the patients for a few minutes at a time, and the rest of the hours were spent talking and sharing our stories. Families would talk about their journeys, what worked and what didn't, and how they managed the stress of caring for their spouse or child. Some of the group had been to other clinics in the area, and they told me about the ones they had tried and what had worked for their loved ones.

One clinic in particular stuck out to us, and so we decided to look into it. The Hoxsey Biomedical Center was also in Tijuana, and was known for providing all-natural, alternative treatments for cancer. One such treatment involved a one-day appointment where they would review your blood work and labs and create a specialized tonic made of natural herbs. The Hoxsey tonic has been around since the early 1900s, and has produced an astonishing amount of positive results in cancer patients. I called and made an appointment for Lenny on his day off from treatments, and a few days later we had a bottle of herbal tonic made to help Lenny's body detoxify and normalize cell metabolism. We stowed it away in our bags to take home with us and use once Lenny had finished his current treatments.

By far the most difficult part of the entire trip was being so far away from Jordan and the rest of our family. After about two and half weeks in Mexico, Jordan was missing us to the point that I decided to fly home for a week to be with him. I took the tonic back with me so that we would know it was safe at home, and I headed to Virginia. I spent eight days with Jordan and we had a blast. On the eighth morning, Jordan said, "Mom, I'm good now. You go back and be with dad until it's time to come home."

Since neither Jordan nor Lenny liked the idea of having Jordan come back to Tijuana with me, he asked if he could go down to Charlotte to stay with Diana and her husband. I booked my flight to Mexico out of Charlotte and the next morning we drove down to North Carolina. Saying goodbye, again, was difficult, but I was also missing Lenny terribly by this point and so by the tenth day home, I was on my way back to Tijuana.

The following week, Lenny was scheduled to have his first PET scan to determine how thoroughly his body was responding to treatment. The PET scans were done at a local hospital, but getting there required a trip by bus through Tijuana. He received his contrast and then was called in for his scan. In the waiting room, I began to notice the facility around me. I was sitting in a state-of-the-art hospital, clean and modern, and on the walls were painted beautiful scriptures. I could have been in a hospital anywhere in the world. After a few hours of waiting, Lenny emerged with his images and we headed back to the clinic.

Not long after we walked through the clinic doors, Lenny started shaking uncontrollably with chills and a high fever. I tried to be calm, but I was panicking on the inside. Up until that point, he had not experienced any adverse reaction to the treatments apart from fatigue. Out of nowhere he spiked a fever which eventually reached 105 degrees, despite the nurses best efforts to bring it down. We went back and forth, putting ice cold compresses on his forehead and eventually, nearly two hours later, his fever gradually dropped. The only logical explanation was that Lenny had an allergic reaction to the contrast that was put in his body for the PET scan. Once he completed that day's round of therapies and had a night to rest, he looked good as new.

While we waited for the scan results to be translated from Spanish into English, we had an opportunity to celebrate with other patients at the clinic who received clear scans. Even those who had only a small amount of improvement were supported and celebrated.

Any progress was good progress. It meant there was hope.

On Thursday of our final week in Mexico, Lenny was called in to review his scan results with Dr. Bautista, the Godfather. In the six weeks of treatment, the tumor shrunk by more than half its size and decreased in density. The SUV on his scan was 7.5%, an incredible improvement from the last scan he had back home. Dr. Bautista was optimistic and encouraged Lenny to stay another three to four weeks, encouraging him that the tumor could be completely gone in that amount of time.

The thought of staying to see if further treatment would help was tempting, but Lenny was ready to go home and carry on with treatments as best he could on his own. Saying goodbye to the people we had met at the clinic was challenging—we had been part of each other's fight and journey, something that cannot be replicated or replaced. We decided to create a Facebook group to stay in touch and follow-up with each other on progress and healing. We shared hugs and photos and contact information, thanked the doctors and nurses and got on our last shuttle back to California.

Apart from gaining friends and community, we gained a lot of information during our stay in Mexico. Lenny and I researched the various machines that were used in his therapy and made a list of the ones we would get once we were back home: the Rife machine, heat therapy machine, and a magnetic bed. All of these were things he could add to his daily routine, and all of them had played a part in his progress at the clinic.

We felt rich with information and a renewed sense of purpose.

We left the clinic that day with a list of supplements, one of the vaccines that had been part of Lenny's therapy, and a list of approved foods and recipes from chef Raul. We also left with an enormous amount of hope.

CHAPTER TWELVE

It Is Well with Our Souls

Lenny and I landed in Charlotte and were greeted at the airport by Jordan and Diana. They swept us back to Diana's house where her husband, Tristan, had dinner waiting for us, and we spent the evening filling them in on our time in Mexico and the hopeful results of Lenny's scans. They laughed as we shared the adventures—and misadventures— of trying to navigate a foreign country where neither of us spoke the language. As we sat together, I felt an immense gratitude for these people I get to call family. They, too, had been down a difficult road of navigating life with cancer. This journey was theirs as much as it was ours.

When we finally arrived home in Virginia, I passionately launched into my new role as Lenny's personal chef. Lenny was going to immediately begin using the Hoxsey tonic, which required he restrict his diet even more than what we had grown accustomed to at the Mexico clinic.

We removed tomato products and vinegar from his diet, along with all processed sugar, gluten, soy and dairy. Everything we purchased was non-GMO and organic, and I religiously read all nutrition labels to ensure there weren't any hidden ingredients. I quickly learned that the number one ingredient, in even the most unlikely of foods, was sugar. It was everywhere. I also learned why so many health programs recommend shopping the perimeter of the grocery store. Almost every pre-packaged item I picked up had added sugar, among other things.

I resorted to purchasing certain products online and the rest at local grocery stores. Shopping for healthy food reminded me of the huge monetary burden that cancer—or any illness—has on families. In a matter of minutes, I spent over $600 on Amazon, just on food and spices. It's estimated that nationally in 2017, over $14 billion was spent on the care and treatment of lymphoma alone.[20] That doesn't include any other type of cancer, and it doesn't include supplements, diet, or alternative treatment expenses or even lost income due to an inability to work. While $14 billion is an incredible amount of money, on the other side of that number is a category of patient who isn't spending money on lymphoma.

A huge number of people don't take prescribed medications or treatments because they simply can't afford them.

[20] https://progressreport.cancer.gov/after/economic_burden

The trip to Mexico, with its three week extension, ended up costing us our savings that we had intended to put into a new house. Another $27,000 was put on credit cards in order to purchase the Rife machine, magnetic infrared mat and a few other machines like the ones Lenny had used at the clinic. Regardless of the cost, we considered ourselves incredibly fortunate to have the money to pour into Lenny's health.

Our living room quickly became a mini-wellness center, which included Lenny's far infrared sauna and the new gadgets we had learned about in Mexico. Meals became an experiment in the art of cooking with unfamiliar ingredients—and getting my teenager to like what I cooked. We adjusted, though, and this new lifestyle became easier for all of us as time went on. Lenny was so gracious with my recipes and seemed to enjoy what I was able to concoct. Jordan was still hesitant, and so some nights he and I would have a different meal altogether, leaving Lenny to enjoy my non-GMO, gluten free, organic creations.

Our first visit to Dr. Alberico quickly reminded us that we were no longer in Mexico. He was incredibly positive about Lenny's results, and for that we were grateful. Dr. Alberico was always an advocate for health and wellness. When we shared about the different treatments Lenny had undergone in Mexico, however, he was completely unfamiliar with almost all of them. He was familiar with immunotherapy, but I later discovered that some of the newest cancer drugs on the market are labeled "Immunotherapy" drugs, simply because they work by binding to a certain protein on T-lymphocytes, the immune system's cancer fighting cells. The drug prevents cancer cells from binding to that same protein, therefore allowing the T-lymphocytes to do their job. While this type of immunotherapy seems to be effective in certain cancer patients, there is still a litany of side effects similar to chemotherapy, including the potential for the immune system to turn on itself and attack the other organs in the body.

These new immunotherapy drugs can cost upwards of $100,000 a year for treatments, but in some scenarios they are being hailed as the cancer treatment drugs of the future. So far in 2018, the FDA has already approved a melanoma drug that will cost $141,000 for just 12 weeks of treatment.[21] If these drugs really could save or extend someone's life, why on earth are they so inaccessible? I left the oncologist's office that day completely frustrated with our society's inability to marry conventional and alternative medicine.

If there are options available to people, both natural and pharmaceutical, we should be doing everything in our power to help people find and afford the treatments that could save them.

Instead, we have FDA approved drugs that cost hundreds of thousands, and natural supplements and treatments that are affordable, but either illegal in the United States or unavailable through insurance.

---

[21] https://www.drugwatch.com/news/2015/10/07/cost-of-cancer/

Lenny's next scans were scheduled for the following December, and so, in the meantime, we threw ourselves into our new lifestyle. With the depletion of our savings, our plans to build a new home were put on hold. Instead, we turned our current little ranch house into the London Wellness Center, and every day Lenny invested in eating well, taking his Hoxsey tonic, and using his machines. Our goal and our mission endured, to make Lenny well.

Not long after we had returned from Mexico, one of Lenny's business partners approached him about our planned home-build. He asked Lenny how much we needed to complete the project. Lenny thought it through and told his partner that he could get the property and build the house with $100,000. His partner looked at him and said, "Consider it done. We will loan you the money. You guys need a break."

Lenny came home that evening overjoyed and overwhelmed by his partner's generosity. I remembered the trip to Disney back in the early days of Lenny's fight, and again felt humbled and grateful for the extreme generosity of other people. Even when we fail to see it, there is goodness and love all around us. We experienced it in seemingly small moments, like someone showing up at our door with a pizza, to the company of friends in the hospital, at the Mexico clinic, and now the gift of a loan that would allow us to rebuild pieces of what had previously been lost. Surely this is what the goodness of God looks like on this earth.

We began construction just a few months later and within a year of returning from Mexico, we were settled into our new home. Lenny's scans, in the midst of the building project, revealed that his tumor had shrunk another 16% since we returned from

Mexico and began our in-home wellness clinic. Between April and December, he experienced a total of over 66% reduction in the abdominal tumor. We knew we were doing something right.

In Mexico we had celebrated even the smallest victories with the other patients, and so we made that our practice at home as well. We would celebrate even the slightest change or decrease in the cancer growth, even if the conventional medical world looked at us with pity, not wanting to breed false hope.

If hope really is from God, then it can't possibly be false.

Hope became our way of life and our prayer: "May the God of hope fill you with all joy and peace as you trust in him, so that you may overflow with hope by the power of the Holy Spirit" (Romans 15:13). I thought that maybe our home should have its own sign: "Miracles Happen Here."

Lenny's next scans, in 2018, showed mixed results. We were taken aback, but we refused to get back on the rollercoaster and most of all, we refused to give in to fear or doubt. Dr. Alberico recommended Lenny start taking Keytruda, which was recently approved by the FDA to treat NHL. It was previously tested for lung cancer, and approved a few years ago to treat a specific type of that disease. However, this new "immunotherapy" has been rapidly approved for several different types of cancers, and most recently blood related cancers such as NHL. Much like the other immunotherapy drugs, it can cost up to $150,000 per year, with a recommended 24-month treatment plan.

Lenny declined the Keytruda, determining that the side effects listed were actually worse than the side effects of chemotherapy. How strange that we vilify options like cannabis oil and Hoxsey tonic, make B17 illegal and worry about people taking herbal remedies that could supposedly harm them, but we are happy to promote a drug that can turn your own immune system against you. We deny access to the most natural, readily available ingredients, but why? Why are we so afraid to give people options? Why are we okay with denying people a true choice?

We will always be grateful to Dr. Alberico and the other oncologists for helping Lenny combat his cancer over the years, and for providing treatment options when he needed them most. At this point, we truly believe that diet, attitude and belief play the largest role in the overall health of the cancer patient. My hope is that the conventional medical world would begin to see this and point people toward wellness—in whatever form— and not just a pharmaceutical. All of the alternative methods that Lenny pursued over the years have profoundly helped his immune system, even allowing it to sustain the harsh effects of chemotherapy and radiation.

While we couldn't always gauge the physical effect of our alternative choices, the times of longest remission for Lenny were when he chose to do the radical, alternative treatments over the conventional ones.

Had we been aware of some of the alternative therapies from the beginning, he may have been able to avoid chemotherapy altogether.

Above all else, every choice we made—whether made in pain and fear, or hope and faith—brought us further along on a journey that always had one destination: Lenny's healing. The road has brought us through 17 years of trial and error, highs and lows, but it is not over. The unknown is still in front of us, but we approach it now with security and hope. I believe we can confidently say, it is well with our souls.

CHAPTER THIRTEEN

The Greatest of These Is Love

As I sit writing this, nearly 17 years have passed since Lenny was first diagnosed with Non-Hodgkins Lymphoma. I look back at those early days and don't know whether I should laugh or cry at our pure innocence, drive, and utter disregard for the status quo of the cancer world. There were moments in our process when Lenny and I felt completely opposed to conventional cancer treatments, convinced ourselves we would not use them, and then succumbed to what was available in our moment of need. Some may see it as fickle, I think it is the reality of desperation.

From those first devastating moments in the hospital in 2001, to the complete acceptance and unashamed hope at the clinic in Mexico in 2017, our lives have been held together by one simple and divine truth: love. We had the love of our families and friends, our desperate and unwavering love for one another, and we had the love of God—perhaps what some would consider the least tangible of all.

But for us, it was God's love that upheld everything else.

Just prior to Lenny's second round of chemotherapy treatments, and his eventual stem cell transplant, I was reminded of this love through the gift of my three-day retreat, the Walk to Emmaus. During the retreat, we were encouraged to write a letter to ourselves. While this may seem a strange practice—the act of trying to encourage yourself as though you were on the outside of your life looking in—it had a profound impact on my perspective. In fact, it resulted in providing a tool that I wish I had with me from the beginning. After the retreat, I returned to that letter over and over again, seeking comfort, hope, and the courage to keep going.

My dearest Andrea,

Stop beating yourself up. It's not your fault. Give yourself a hug. God loves you and you are worthy to be loved. He forgives you. You are the apple of His eye.

It is short and simple, but I read and re-read that letter over 200 times in the days and weeks that followed. In recent years there has been a resurgence of interest in self-care and people seeking to understand the role it plays in our overall well-being.

With the epidemic of depression in our society and culture, helping people know how to combat self-destructive thoughts and feelings is more important than ever. As we try to understand the importance of self-care, we also are trying to understand what it looks like. Prayer, meditation, and exercise are some of the most commonly promoted practices for taking care of oneself. For others, implementing affirmations as a daily routine has proven not only helpful, but also empowering.

For me, this letter serves as an affirmation, a reminder that I am okay, I am loved, and I am covered by a God who I may not be able to see, but whose love and influence I experience all around me.

Love is not an intangible, unattainable experience. In fact, it is ours to give and receive as easily and freely as we choose.

Despite the most challenging moments in our lives, it is sometimes the simplest act of love that brings us closer to knowing and understanding both God and ourselves.

When my dad passed away, it was my job to make the arrangements for his funeral, which meant sorting through old photos, creating a slideshow and designing a program for the day. A new friend, someone who I had only just met, stepped in and helped me take care of all the little details. I hardly knew her, and yet there she was, willing to offer her time in a moment of need.

Our lives are sprinkled with these experiences of support from both complete strangers and from our closest family. In the midst of chaos or struggle, it is easy to feel overwhelmed or burdened by the good intentions of other people, which is why the tangible and unexpected acts of others speaks so loudly to our broken souls. Tickets to Disney World, dinner for our family, flowers in the hospital, cake on our birthdays—these were some of the most tangible encounters with love that we experienced. When I look back, I can see the impact of every expression of support in our lives. Family astounded us with their willingness to give in whatever way possible. Lenny's sister organized the fundraiser early on to pay for some of the alternative medicine and Diana designed a t-shirt that read, "Team London" and raised $3000 toward our medical expenses.

When Lenny and I decided to go to the clinic in Mexico, a decision that was made over a period of just a few short weeks, some friends of ours reached out in the midst of that decision and paid for our airfare to and from San Diego. It can be difficult to receive from others when they choose to reach out with generosity. We minimize our need, or how deserving we are of such a gift. In truth, the greatest thing we can do for ourselves and the person giving is to express the reality of our gratitude.

Generosity is an act of love, and we are all deserving of love—always.

This was profoundly demonstrated to me and Lenny while we were in Mexico. As we shared meals and stories with the other patients and their families, we became aware of how much these people—ourselves included—needed to be reminded of their value.

When we understand our worth, our place in this world and the unique value we bring to it—we suddenly have a purpose to keep fighting.

If our presence on this earth is pointless, just a great cosmic accident, then what are we fighting for? Why do we want so desperately to live, love, and be known?

While Lenny and I find our inspiration in different places—his anthem is 80's rock and roll while mine is the latest tune on K-love—our motivation is the same: to know love and share that love with others. One of my favorite scriptures is a letter that the Apostle Paul wrote to the church in Corinth sometime between AD 53 and 57. Through nearly two thousand years of history and translations, the words have impacted my life. The well- known 13th chapter is read at weddings around the world, and while it is easy to swipe the words aside, I can't help but let the depth of their truth influence my life. Paul wrote that without love, there is nothing. We can give away our belongings, we can accomplish the greatest feats of strength or wisdom, we can live a successful, rich life, but without love, it will all be pointless.

Sitting in the worn out clinic in Mexico, we did our best to share love with those around us. We shared our fight and our drive to find a solution that would work. Lenny joked with other patients and did everything possible to pass on his positive attitude and encourage everyone to keep fighting. After returning home, we did our best to stay in touch with the other families through email and social media.

Our purpose and our goal was to simply love as best we could.

We knew what it was like to need support and belief, and all we could do was hope what we offered was enough to help even just a little.

Once we were back in Virginia, we found out that one of the young men that Lenny met at the clinic eventually lost his battle with cancer. His mom, who we had grown close with during our time in Mexico, sent Lenny all of her son's unused alternative treatments shortly after her son passed away. We were overwhelmed that she would think of Lenny in her time of deepest grief. That is a love that goes beyond understanding.

A short time later, we received a card from another family we had met in Mexico. Their 17-year old son also lost his battle with cancer and we felt the grief of his family. On the outside of the card was a picture of a man running through the mountains with the words "Don't Quit" at the top. Underneath was an inscription of 2 Corinthians 12:9, "My grace is sufficient for you, for My power is made perfect in weakness." The words of the card encouraged us to not quit, to lean on God's grace and remember that we can all make a difference in the midst of our own battle no matter how hopeless things look. Even in pain, this mother took the time to send us her encouragement. "Dear Andrea and Lenny, The message on the front of this card is what you taught me," she wrote. "[My son] died with his family around him. He died peacefully and gently. We held his hand and kissed his precious head. We told him of our love and how much God loved him...God is good, and we are so grateful to you, Andrea and Lenny, for walking this beautiful walk of faith with us."

We wept for this sweet mother and the loss she and her family endured. We have shed tears for many who have come into our lives and then been taken away again far too soon. Nothing can prepare you for the gaping hole that is left when a loved one departs from this life. Whether taken unexpectedly or after a long, difficult fight, the pain of loss remains the same.

But in these moments of overwhelming grief, we can still taste the thread of love that winds its way throughout our lives.

There is a song I often played while working out or in my moments of prayer that spoke to the chaos of our lives. "Praise You in This Storm" by Casting Crowns was a constant reminder of what it means to believe in something bigger than ourselves— whether we call that thing God or love—even in the midst of life's burdens. In my depression and my fight with anger, I would often question God, challenge Him and His greater purpose or supposed plan for our lives.

This song would remind me that circumstances change, but love and God are unchanging. He is the constant in the midst of an inconsistent reality.

Lenny's undeniable positivity proved to be the greatest example of love throughout our wild journey. The man whose body was fighting to survive, the one who stood on ground zero with cancer and waged war against a disease that has overrun our world, he was a constant source of laughter and joy for our family and I thank the Lord every day for his presence in our lives. We might think that to talk about the love of God and presence of miracles is to talk about things that are "supernatural" and intangible. My family, my children and my husband are the most tangible expression of God's love for me. Lenny is my miracle, a gift from a Father who cares about my life enough to bring me a partner who loves and cares for me. I only hope that I can return that love.

Lenny reminds me often, in small ways and in his ever-constant drive to keep living, that what we have to offer those around us is a taste of the love that has blessed our lives so profoundly. For us, the source is and always will be a loving God, the creator of all things. For some, the understanding of love is based solely in the tangible expression of goodness around them. Regardless of where you encounter it, I pray that you also will experience the sustaining power of love in your life. Lenny and I bless you to experience the truth and beauty of love in the midst of your own unique journey. It is the greatest gift we have to offer one another.

"And now these three remain: faith, hope and love. But the greatest of these is love" (1 Corinthians 13:13).

A Letter from Lenny

Dear Reader,

I'd like to first start off by saying how fortunate I am to have found this amazing woman, Andrea, who has literally kept me alive. I know that I would not be here if our paths had not crossed.

God had a plan, it wasn't my plan and I'm sure it wasn't Andrea's plan. Yes, at times it has been difficult but somehow, someway, we have persevered through all the madness.

The thought of putting our life all together in a book has been on her heart for a long while.

Andrea and I kept thinking there would be an ending to all this cancer but then there would be another chapter. I applaud my wife for seeing this book become a reality. My heart is full.

Presumably anyone diagnosed with cancer, the first thing that goes through your mind is "why Me?" I tried to answer that question and figure out why the cancer cells activated in my body. As far as I could tell, I was always a healthy person. I had a pretty good diet, or so I thought. I worked out and I stayed fit, and growing up I avoided the drugs and the binge drinking that so many others were participating in. So why me?

I also had my family to consider. Telling them about my diagnosis was incredibly difficult. All I could think about was, *I have cancer, there is no cure and I'm going to die.* My mind just kept going to what the doctor said, "You have seven to nine years to live with this." When we traveled up to NVA to tell my family, who had all gathered at my sister's house, I tried to stay strong but could see the fear in everyone's eyes and Andrea had to step in to finish explaining. It was a pretty low moment.

Eventually, I got angry with the disease and I wanted to take action. Instead of pitying myself, I wanted to do whatever it would take to fight—and beat—cancer.

There were several things that helped me overcome my mental battle.

I had the support of my wife, my family, and my closest friends. My best friend Vance would challenge me to keep going. "Get your mind right," he would say.

"Stay strong." I would workout, because that felt like something real that I could do for myself. I would take my frustration out on the weights and listen to some good music while I got my mind straight and focused on the things I needed to overcome.

When my youngest son, Jordan, was born, it was a fresh reminder of my desire to live and raise my family. At first, I asked myself if I would even be there to watch my son grow up. And then other questions started bombarding me. Who is going to fill in and be the father role? Who is going to teach him all the things that he needs to know to become a man? I hated feeling like he would have to live with this his whole life—we tried to shield him as best we could.

Our older kids were upset when they heard the diagnosis, and did their best to understand what was happening, but they were also still young. We tried to make family life as normal and functional as possible. When the economy crashed and we were fighting to pay for treatments and put a roof over our heads, we had to sacrifice certain things that felt normal to us as a family. But we still did our best to maintain connection and live life to the fullest. While we tried to create a normal and healthy life for our kids, the awareness of cancer never really left me or Andrea, we always knew it was there. We always had test results to look at, and we were constantly critiquing and changing something in our lifestyle. It never leaves your mind. Even in remission, it is always back there somewhere.

The battle in the mind is ongoing and so keeping a positive outlook and a mindset that I would overcome was a continual process. When I was first diagnosed, there were no conventional treatments available to me, so pursuing alternative options made sense. The first alternative treatment I tried worked, and my swollen lymph nodes went back to their normal size. That relieved a lot of the hysteria in my mind. When you visibly see something that actually works, you take on an entirely new outlook on what it means to beat cancer.

One of the hardest decisions for me over the years to come, was saying "no" to the chemotherapy, radiation and other conventional treatments that my oncologist, who is obviously a extremely educated and accomplished physician offered me.

As the years passed, sometimes a different question would invade my mind. We read or see stories of cancer everyday or watch TV and learn that someone else is dying of cancer. After awhile, the question became, *why am I still here?* When I went to Mexico, and we were doing their treatments, I realized that the patients who seemed to do better—physically and emotionally— were the ones pursuing the alternative options. It dawned on me, through meeting all these different people, that if I hadn't done any of the alternative stuff, I probably still wouldn't be here. I'm thankful everyday that I did the sauna, the better eating habits, and the supplements from the earliest days of my diagnosis.

As the years have gone by, I realized that we can help a lot of people by sharing what we have walked through and the things we have tried.

While I have seen a lot of things positively impact my body, Andrea and I are still looking for the alternate solution that heals—the thing that we can say with certainty can heal cancer 100%. In the meantime, there are so many things that have helped reduce symptoms, shrink tumors, and assist in both my longevity and quality of life. A lot of those things are listed in the resource section that follows, but these are some of the things I would highly recommend:

» Find a competent alternative doctor. Get as many opinions as you need, but seek alternative opinions from people who have had consistent good results.

» Get extensive blood panels done right away. These are different than traditional blood tests and will tell you what is really going on inside of your body. (Live blood cell analysis and blood tests that reveal any inflammation in the body as well as deficiencies in certain nutrients).

» Get on the supplements your body is lacking (a lot of people are deficient in vitamin D3 as well as many others, do your research)

» The Terry Natural brand is recommended by many alternative health practitioners and I like these three in particular: Curamed 750 (Cucurmin), Bosmed 500 (frankincense), Clinical OPC (grape seed).

» Radically change your diet. We were meant to eat whole foods, not chemically altered and processed foods. Along with this comes changing your lifestyle, sleep patterns, what you eat, the times you eat and the amount of water you drink. Eat in balance and get a good night's sleep and fast overnight. This helps the body to heal because it's not working overtime to digest foods while sleeping.

» Research. Begin researching different options and methods that are a good fit for you because there are no "one size fits all" healing methods.

» Mentally you must keep your mind focused on positive things and not always focusing on the disease. I did this by focusing on designing my family's dream home while sitting at our kitchen table practically every night for two years. We were able to eventually build it and we live in that very home today.

Whether you choose to go through alternative treatments or conventional treatments (I did both), there are things you can do today to help your body fight cancer.

If you do choose to go through traditional treatment, it is not recommended that you take alternative medicines at the same time. When you are getting whacked with chemo, for example, the cocktail is destroying everything in your body. The idea behind alternative medicine is to rebuild your body and boost your immune system. By doing this during chemo, sometimes the cancer gets rebuilt in the process. Instead, the best thing you can do for yourself during chemo and radiation is to eat clean, avoid sugar and processed foods, and don't use the alternative medicines until you are done with traditional treatments.

A lot of people are using the CBD oil for pain and sleep, and a lot of people are doing THC as well. This is a great option during both conventional and alternative treatments if your body can tolerate it. There is a Facebook group that Andrea and I discovered that has been especially helpful: Cannabis Oil Success

Stories. It's a great community with a lot of information for those just starting their journey and those looking for a new option.

One thing I have learned over the past 17 years is that we cannot take this life for granted. Every time we went to the traditional doctor, I would feel the pressure of time and my mind would get all tangled up in the fear of cancer, of leaving life too soon and it was frustrating. My clock is in front of me and my expiration date could be around the corner. There was so much I didn't—and couldn't—know. It was overwhelming.

That is why mindset is such an important part of the journey of overcoming. What are you living for? What are you fighting for? The love of God and my family have played such a huge role in my positive outlook on life. I am surrounded by people who will fight for me and alongside me, who pray for my healing and celebrate with me when there is victory of any size.

Andrea and I are still constantly researching, looking for new ways to beat cancer and not just keep it at bay. We are always making new discoveries—alternative practitioners with an enthusiasm for the latest research. There is Essiac tea (made in Canada) which uses cancer fighting herbs, the Hoxsey tonic that we discovered in Mexico, just to name a few. The search continues as we seek to discover a method that will bring complete healing, the missing piece to the puzzle we've been putting together for years. We also found that *The truth about Cancer* documentary which can be found online, is another awesome source of information and validated a lot of what we are doing to fight cancer.

We wrote this book not just to share our story and our research, but because we know how difficult it can be to ask for help in the midst of battling a disease or a struggle of any kind. No one should have to battle alone, so even if we never meet you, it is my hope that this book will help you find hope, inspiration to try new things and find new options, and even just the knowledge that you are not alone in this fight.

If I can give you anything, I hope it is the patience to endure and the motivation to keep going. Trying to get your body to its optimal health is a journey. Some treatments that are available, like chemo and radiation, are a quick fix to destroy cancer cells in the body and unfortunately, healthy cells too. But it doesn't go away overnight. Regardless of the method, it takes time and endurance to walk yourself back to both physical and emotional health. Andrea and I are still learning, evolving treatment methods that work for us, and doing our best to find peace and enjoy life in the middle of a battle.

If we can do it, so can you.

Stay strong. Continue to fight the good fight. We will win this war together.

Sincerely,
Jack "Lenny" London

RESOURCES

As I sat down to compile a list of all of the resources and products we recommend, I realized there has been so much we have found beneficial over the past seventeen years. Lenny and I decided to share with you the products we have found to be the most helpful, including the things that Lenny remains using to this day.

Since the very beginning we have consistently gleaned information from many sources—doctors, alternative practitioners, online resources, and books—and we strongly believe that while there are many things that can contribute to cancer growth, there are three main contributing elements that are completely controllable: stress, diet, and mouth health.

Oral health plays a key role in maintaining an overall healthy body. When Lenny was first diagnosed back in 2001, he had recently undergone a major root canal. The alternative doctor advised Lenny to have the tooth pulled in order to prevent any infection. Your mouth health can reveal larger issues in the body, and alternately, a weakened immune system can mean greater risk of oral infection or other diseases. With improved oral health, a change of diet, daily supplements, and a small amount of alternative medicine, Lenny's 23 swollen lymph nodes returned to normal in less than six months. This was accomplished without any conventional medicine.

Diet, another controllable health factor, is particularly significant in the United States where much of the food we eat has been genetically modified and tampered with in a way that no longer provides our bodies with the nutrients we need. A clean, organic and non-GMO diet is the key to a healthier body: a body that can fight disease.

Cancer loves sugar and an acidic environment. Every food that we eat or drink can be placed into two categories: foods that strengthen the cancer cells and/or the microbes in the cancer cells, and foods that contain the nutrients needed to assist the immune system in killing cancer cells. Examples of foods that assist cancer growth are refined sugar, refined flour, soda, meats, trans fats, and dairy products. These foods not only aid cancer cell growth but also cause inflammation in the body, inhibiting the immune system from focusing on killing the cancer cells.

Non-inflammatory and alkaline foods that help the body maintain balance and help strengthen the immune system include purple grapes (with seeds and skin intact), red raspberries with seeds, strawberries with seeds, broccoli, cauliflower, herbs, carrots, pineapples, almonds, and beans. Neither of these lists are exhaustive, simply a sampling of what we have learned throughout seventeen years of research and through the process of elimination.

Lenny eats a clean, gluten free, sugar free and non- GMO diet. We also purchase organic items whenever they are available to us. This diet may sound boring and restrictive, but Lenny has grown to enjoy the foods I make for him. At the end of this section we have included a list of the key foods we purchase—plus how we make these items budget-friendly—as well as some of Lenny's favorite recipes. Some of these foods we learned about in Mexico. The clinic provided an on-site chef who prepared all the meals for the patients. While Lenny was there, receiving treatment and eating a clean diet, his tumor shrank 50% in only six weeks.

We consider our supplements to be part of our diet, and therefore the expense to be part of our food bill. For us, supplements are not an option, but a necessity. Over the years, we have found some of the most superb supplements through different network marketing companies. A lot of times these companies spend the bulk of their money on product research, development, and manufacturing—rather than marketing and advertising—since their marketing is accomplished through the network of resellers. While we recommend you do your research before partnering with a network marketing company (and their product), we have come to see the benefits of this approach, both financially and as it pertains to finding the highest quality products. Because our supplement purchases are attached to a business, we are able to use tax write offs for a lot of our expenses. We save money while helping others get healthy and find a potential additional source of income, which makes it a win for everyone involved.

The final controllable lifestyle factor is stress. When unmanaged, stress can inhibit your body's ability to fight disease. It can cause a weakened immune system and an emotional environment that depletes your body of energy. Lenny's stress management techniques include working out, spending time with friends and family, and maintaining an overall positive outlook on life. Everyone is different in their methods, so finding what helps you manage stress and stay positive will be key to your body's overall health.

Below we have outlined several different resources we feel are worth sharing includingfood, recipes, supplements, alternative therapies, and alternative practitioners/clinics. While some of the products and practices we recommend may seem pricey, we have figured out that all the alternative methods cost just about the same as getting two CT scans per year and paying regular copayments. In fact, in order to help with the cost of living a healthy lifestyle, we recently discovered a facility in our area (but outside of our healthcare network) that offers CT scans at a much more affordable price. While the facility is local to Virginia (www.mri-ct.com), there may be similar options available near you. By using this facility, we are saving approximately $7,000 per year. We now use that money for Lenny and our family to have some of the best foods and supplements on the market.

We long for the day when conventional medicine can be combined with alternative treatment, and the medical world makes the much-needed decision to treat the patient with a more holistic approach: healing the body, mind and spirit. We believe this is the way of the future and we truly hope that our story has given you inspiration and hope to keep moving forward no matter what your diagnosis or prognosis. In addition to listening to what your doctors recommend, it is our hope that you also take your health into your own hands by researching other options that are available to you. We pray that no matter what method(s) you choose, you find healing and hope on your journey.

Food

The listed foods are the items that we always have in the house. We compare prices in our local grocery store to amazon.com. With a Prime membership and free two-day shipping, sometimes buying online ends up being the more affordable option.

Produce (Organic)

» Garlic (Spice World brand)
» Leeks
» Onions
» Bell peppers
» Broccoli
» Green beans
» Spinach
» Asparagus
» Red potatoes
» Lemons
» Oranges
» Berries
» Bananas
» Fresh herbs

Miscellaneous (organic whenever possible)

- » Bragg's Liquid Aminos
- » Olive oil
- » Coconut oil
- » Agave
- » Stevia
- » Sea salt
- » Black pepper
- » Brown rice
- » Sugar-free and gluten-free Pizza crust by Namaste Foods
- » Gluten-free baking and pancake mix by Pamela
- » Gluten-free brown rice pasta and lasagna by Tinkyada
- » Lentils
- » Split peas
- » Dairy-free cheese
- » Coconut milk
- » Plant-based protein powder
- » Alkaline filtered water from glass bottles

Recipes

We eat fresh vegetables daily and only one to two servings of fruits mainly to keep the natural sugar intake low. I cook almost everything with olive oil, garlic, lemons and onions. These are a few of Lenny's favorite recipes for inspiration.

Pizza

Crust:

>> Namaste Foods organic gluten free pizza crust. Make the crust as directed on the package. Bake for 20 minutes and then brush with olive oil.

Toppings/Sauce:

>> Sauté garlic, onions and peppers in olive oil

>> Add cubed organic chicken

>> Pour topping mixture onto pre-baked crust

>> Add organic Daya non-dairy cheese and a small handful of organic parmesan

>> Bake an additional 15 minutes or cheese is melted

Organic Stir Fry

>> Prepare organic brown rice

>> While rice is cooking, sauté organic onions, peppers, and garlic in olive oil

>> Add organic chicken and organic spices of choice.

>> Cook until done

>> Add a few tablespoons of liquid aminos

>> Pour entire mixture over brown rice

Shrimp Scampi

» Wild caught shrimp

» Organic garlic

» Olive oil

» Fresh herbs (parsley, basil and thyme)

» Organic butter (1/4 stick)

» Gluten-free spaghetti

Sauté the garlic and shrimp in olive oil. Add the herbs and butter to the pan and stir until melted. Toss shrimp and herb mixture with gluten free spaghetti noodles. Sprinkle with organic parmesan (This is optional. Dairy should be eliminated from the diet so we only use very little amounts of cheese and butter.)

Green Smoothie

» 1-2 cups organic spinach

» Handful of berries

» Banana

» 1 scoop organic plant-based protein powder

» Organic unsweetened coconut milk

» Crushed ice

» Blend well

Pancakes

» Pamela's gluten-free pancake mix

» Add water and organic egg

» Use coconut or olive oil for nonstick

» Top with fruit or organic agave instead of syrup

Supplements

» B-17 500mg (apricotpower.com)

» B-15 100 mg (apricotpower.com)

» CuraMed 750 mg (Terry Naturally)

» OPC 400mg (Terry Naturally)

» Bosmed with boswellia 500mg (Terry Naturally)

» CoQ10 (Life Extension)

» Vitamin D3 (NOW)

» Digestive Enzymes (NOW)

» Probiotics (NOW)

» Montana Yew tip capsules (Bighorn Botanicals)

» Omegas (Dr. Tobias - drtobias.net)

» Prostate Health (Natural Factors)

» GO energy & CORE AO immune drinks (http://mnetwork.myvoffice.com)

» CBD Hemp Capsules (LivLabs - http://london.livlabsnow.com)

» CBD Hydro Drops (LivLabs - http://london. livlabsnow.com)

» Hoxsey Tonic (Hoxsey Biomedical Center)

» CBD Oil high in THC. (Recipes and more info at http://phoenixtears.ca) There is also a Facebook group called Cannabis Oil Success Stories that has hundreds of testimonies.

» Puréed steamed organic asparagus - 4 tablespoons daily (While this regimen is controversial, Lenny believes it helps so he does it. Search "asparagus fights cancer" to find out more.)

Alternative Treatments (at home)

Lenny uses these therapies to detox his body and relieve stress on a regular basis and the Rife frequencies to combat any active cancer in the body.

» Rife Machine (BCX Ultra from hymbas.com)

» Far Infrared Sauna (healthmatesauna.com)

» Magnetic Heating Mat (by MediCrystal on amazon.com)

Alternative Treatments (at clinic)

Vitamin C infusion. (This is done througha local naturopath. Search "infusion therapy" to find options available in your area.)

DNA testing. (Pamela Wingert - Kankakee Natural Foods. We highly recommend DNA testing on top of normal blood tests and scans. Pamela helps identify what Lenny's body is lacking in terms of diet and supplements, and what frequencies to use for the Rife machine.)

Alternative Clinics

> » Immunity Therapy Center - Tijuana, Mexico
> (immunitytherapycenter.com)

This was the first clinic we visited in Mexico. It was here that Lenny's tumor shrank more than 50% and we discovered the Rife machine, infrared heated mat, and some of our clean eating techniques.

> » Hoxsey Biomedical Center - Tijuana, Mexico
> (hoxseybiomedical.com)

This is where we got the Hoxsey tonic. It is only a one-day appointment. Make sure to bring recent blood work with you if you have it.

TESTIMONIALS

The journey toward Lenny's healing has brought us into contact with many friends, both old and new, who are walking a very similar path. Every story is worth sharing, and here are just two of the many testimonies of waging war on cancer. These two women, our dear friends, have painstakingly put words to their own unique battles and how they have sought to overcome. I hope their stories bless you in the same way their lives have been a blessing to us.

Dawn

When Andrea asked me if I would be interested in writing a bit of my testimony, I was thrilled, honored and immediately said yes. They were headed to Mexico and up the west coast for a family get away, so I had some time. Well that was three months ago and I have struggled so much to get anything onto this paper. So here I am again, no words just type.delete.repeat!

Extramedullary acute myelogenous leukemia/myeloid sarcoma of the small bowel: let's start here! This is the name of the cancer diagnosis I received three years ago. I was told that

I had four months to live if I did not treat it aggressively. The day I heard that diagnosis I heard my heavenly Father so boldly exclaim, "We got this, girl!" as He wrapped this amazing blanket of peace around my entire being.

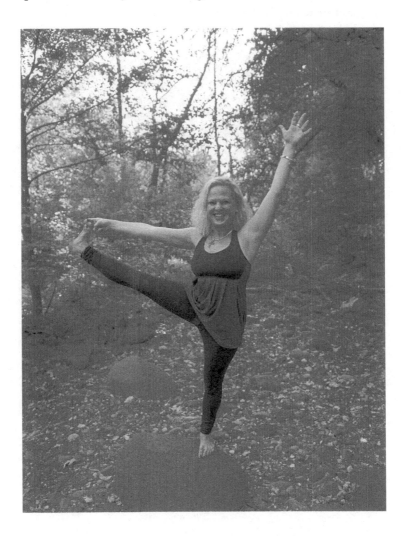

Dawn Kroboth Martinez

I can't say that I was happy that day, or even that I thought I would survive, but I know I was filled with hope. From that point forward, when I prayed, I would say, "Lord, I accept your will for my life. I want to live, and wherever this battle leads me, I will need your peace in my heart to guide me."

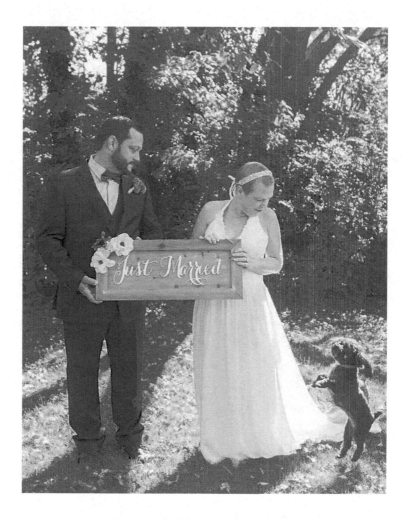

Dawn & Mike wedding day

At the time, I had been working with my father in his tax business for 8 years, studying tax law, taking exams to become an enrolled agent. I was also teaching yoga out of my living room, filling my days with the "good things" in life, and letting Jesus lead me. I had quit smoking, I was eating well, running for fun with my girlfriends on the weekends, volunteering at the church on Sundays, and I had recently "started over" with an ex-boyfriend, Mike. I had a fresh new perspective on love: to be loved and to love unconditionally and with good, healthy boundaries.

It was the end of October and the cool weather had set in. I am energized by 90 degree days and surely could hibernate when the days drop below 75 degrees, but that autumn I was unusually fatigued. I was teaching yoga the coming Monday night and decided Chinese food sounded good, so I grabbed a bite of dinner. Immediately, my stomach started to hurt and I summed it up as a bad choice in food. As the week progressed, I realized it was not the food. With my medical degree—which I obtained while lying on the couch all week reading WebMd—I determined that it had to be the norovirus.

I continued to suffer on my own at home—it was Halloween weekend and I could only imagine what it would be like in an ER. By Sunday night I was doubled over in pain and my stomach was quite distended. Mike finally took me to the ER where a cat-scan showed a blockage in my lower intestines. The doctors determined that they would keep me overnight and wait until Monday morning to have someone review the scan. Since I was not completely blocked, it was not an emergency.

As the surgeon was making his final rounds the next day, he and the head nurse summed up my condition as bad eating habits caused by my western diet: I was inflamed and infected. The surgeon told me they would most likely remove the drain that was relieving the blockage, have me continue on antibiotics, and send me home the following day.

A few short minutes later, the GI doctor came in and asked to speak with me in front of the family. He and his team had reviewed the scans, and he believed I had cancer. This was a radically different diagnosis than the one I had just received from the surgeon. My world was flipped upside down.

Surgery was scheduled for the following morning. They removed a tumor, infected lymph nodes, part of my small intestines, and my appendix. Everything pointed to cancer, but it was unclear what kind until the pathology came back. I was told I would also need a hysterectomy in the future. After the surgery, the oncologist wanted me to start induction chemo right away, but the surgeon thought it would be best to give me two weeks at home to recover.

I spent two weeks at home preparing, but not knowing what I was preparing for. I prayed for a different treatment option, getting on my knees in a messy puddle of tears, pouring out my heart to the One who made me. Because of the unknown path ahead of me, I celebrated Thanksgiving early with loved ones. I was not overly confident about my treatment plan, but I was also too scared not do it. I was one of those people who said I would never do chemo. Never say "never"!

In the midst of following the doctor's orders and his plan to start me on chemo, I also wanted to be proactive and look for alternative options. I immediately started taking a high dose of cannabis oil and I was prepared to use other forms, if needed, to combat pain and nausea. I increased my supplements and added therapeutic grade essential oils to my regimen.

The day I started my induction chemo the sun was shining and it was unusually warm for November. My mom drove me down past the bay before taking me to the hospital. It was gorgeous. The doctors had prepared me for a long stay at the hospital, and they were ready for me when I arrived. They immediately started me on a 23-hour-a-day chemo drip.

The first 72 hours weren't too bad, but that changed rapidly. I remember sitting with my mom in the oncology office, waiting on labs, when the nurse handed me a mask and told me to put it on and go straight home. Do not come in contact with people, she said to me, and if you have a fever over 100.5, go directly to the ER and let them know you are neutropenic. These terms were foreign to me and although I had been handed literature, counseled, and had spoken to many professionals, it was so overwhelming.

On Thanksgiving, when I was supposed to be getting ready for the feast of thanks, I instead experienced a wave of hell that is difficult to describe. I could feel the fever coming on and before I knew it, I was over 104 degrees and the riggers—hardcore chills—had set in. At one point the trauma team came in to my hospital room and I'm pretty sure I thought I was going to die that night.

That day—the wave of hell—was followed by losing every hair on my body, blood transfusions, tests, antibiotics through IV, and another two weeks of fevers. Eventually, my Hysterectomy was scheduled and I was discharged to head up to the Medical College of Virginia in Richmond, about an hour and half from home.

My mom, two sisters, and I rode up to Richmond together. Because they could not find additional cancer in my body, we were thinking this trip was just to confirm that a bone marrow transplant, as originally discussed, would not be necessary, and we would continue with the next scheduled surgery followed by another round of chemo. That was not the case.

At the Medical College, the doctor suggested that my only chance for a cure was to have a bone marrow transplant. He also reminded me that the procedure would require a minimum six-month stay in Richmond. Oh, and my chance of survival was around 20%. What a jerk. The ride home was long, but as we drove, I enjoyed the passing Christmas lights more than usual.

The holidays were filled with so much love and joy, even though I was weak, tired, and my little bald head was cold. My hysterectomy went well, the pathology reports came back clear, and I was cleared by the surgeon to start my next round of chemo. Once again the cycle began.

The day I came home from my chemo round, the Richmond hospital called to let me know that my sisters, who had their bone marrow tested, were not a match. I replied with a simple, "thank you" and then breathed a sigh of relief when I realized God had closed that door. I spent the next two weeks recovering from the chemo, which was not as bad as the first round of treatments, but definitely not a walk in the park.

On February 11th, I was feeling better, hoping to get back to work the following week, when I got a call from the oncologist—I call him Zip. We had a rule that he wasn't allowed to call me before 10 a.m. I am pretty sure he never sleeps, so during chemo he would be at my bedside at 6 a.m., not pleasant for me. Hence the rule to only call after 10. On the phone he was ecstatic and wanted to know if I had talked to anyone from Richmond. He let me know that they had found me a donor in Europe, a 99.9% match, and she had already agreed to move forward with the testing. He said that I would also need to undergo several tests and that I should plan on checking into Richmond on March 14th.

I hung up the phone. My sister was there with me— she had lost a friend years before due to complications of a bone marrow transplant, and although she wanted me to do it, she was scared for me. My mind, my tears, and my mouth were all saying no to the transplant, but my heart was flooded with a peace that I recognized. I knew that peace, it was not mine or the world's, but my Father's, the one I was trusting to heal me. I knew that He was calling me to move forward with the procedure and that His plans for me were good.

My story isn't over, but I have learned so many things throughout the journey. You see, I was that girl that Lenny helped teach how to fight—the one he encouraged before starting chemo. On those days that I felt like I wanted to give up or that I was going to die, I knew that the next day would be better. I held on because I had to, because I could. And I keep holding on—choosing life, so that someday soon, I can share the rest of my story.

Dawn K

Susie

Psalm 139 (paraphrase): I knew you before you were formed in the womb (that secret place). For I am fearfully and wonderfully made.

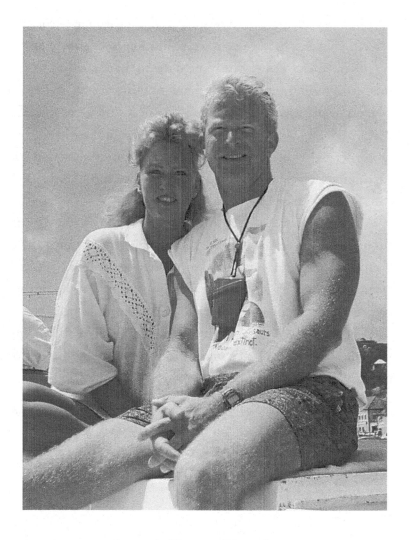

Susie & Tommy Hawthorne

I knew from a very young age that I was adopted. There was no stigma attached to the subject of adoption in my home. It was what it was and I understood that. I knew my birth parents were 16 and 17 and unmarried when they had me. Basically, I was an accident and it was a closed adoption. I grew up with two very loving parents and endured family dysfunction like most families do, knowing I was truly loved. Later, in my adult life, I would have a Mama "A" and a Mama "B."

From childhood through adulthood you will make choices that sometimes have long term consequences. Life is about learning but most importantly, loving and giving. At least that's how I was born to see it.

I was daddy's girl and my dad was my rock and my hero. I adored him. He died in my lap in our backyard from a massive heart attack while we were doing yard work. I was 17 and it was July 17, 1980 at 17:17 military time. And then I wasn't a little princess anymore.

Fast forward through the next ten years, which consisted of lots of trial and error. Add in some anger, unforgiveness, anxiety, PTSD, depression and bitterness from life's bumps and bruises and you have quite a myriad of events that became my story. A brief summary of those ten years included my mother's (Mama "A") nervous breakdown from my father's death, an abortion, two failed marriages due to infidelity and abuse, a brutal sexual assault by a complete stranger and a damaged spirit trying to get by without any type of solid foundation. I was a hot mess.

Soon after, I gave my life to Jesus, met my birth mother, Mama "B," and then met the love of my life: my "all the movie channels man," my hubby.

Both of us came with packaged deals. Mama "A" moved in with me so I could care for her as she faced her first bout with colon cancer. By the way, did I mention, Mama "A" was a narcissist? My husband had two beautiful small children that soon became a part of my soul. We had our hands full, but we were a team and we wanted a second chance at doing this thing called life.

My husband and I got married on February 14, 1998 and two days after returning from our honeymoon, my OBGYN called to inform me that I had an abnormal pap smear.

I listened closely as my OBGYN explained the outpatient procedure I would need to remove the squamous cells that had made their first debut onto my cervix. I was in full understanding of the LEEP procedure explanation but words like "squamous," "precancerous," "ablation," and "HPV" (Human Papillomavirus) weren't sinking in as quickly. My doctor also informed me that should I become pregnant, I would no longer have a cervix to keep the baby secure in my uterus and the probability of being able to carry a baby to full term would be highly unlikely. Doing what I do best, I switched gears to autopilot and successfully endured the surgery. It was the first dance with a beast I would meet with again one day.

"Sing, barren woman,
you who never bore a child;
burst into song, shout for joy,
you who were never in labor;
because more are the children of the desolate woman
than of her who has a husband,"
says the Lord (Isaiah 54:1).

In 2005 I started experiencing abnormal periods and continued follow up appointments with my gynecologist. Another surgical procedure was performed to get the heavy bleeding under control. This procedure consisted of boiling the lining of my uterus away thus completely stopping any outward, monthly blood flow. It was great! No more heavy bleeding. Until one year post surgery. Out of nowhere, I experienced crippling pain in my abdomen. It was so intense at times that I had to lay in a fetal position on the floor in order to get somewhat comfortable. It took a few of these painful attacks before I was back at my gynecologist's office pleading for an explanation.

My doctor performed a pelvic exam and said she would need to "manually dilate" me in order to get a closer look. Not having the slightest clue of what this entailed, I agreed. It wasn't seconds before I was sitting straight up on the examination table sobbing and in a demonic voice instructed her to, "Get this s t out of me." I wanted it gone! If I couldn't conceive then there was no longer a need for the reproductive part of me to stay. I was tired of the pain, problems and reminders from my past.

The surgery was scheduled for October 2006. A complete and total hysterectomy. The incision was from hip bone to hip bone and recovery was tough. Six months post surgery there was still something not quite right. I had pain during intimacy and that had never been an issue before. I went back in to see my gynecologist and we discussed what could be causing the pain. She once again examined and found nothing. Ultrasounds were then ordered and they showed nothing. Dr. B recommended opening me back up for exploratory surgery to see if that would give the answer and so, the surgery date was scheduled. Much to my relief, it was discovered that one of the internal stitches from the hysterectomy had become infected. The stitch was removed and I was now good to go. Finally. No more pain and discomfort. I could put this behind me and go back to comforting my husband who had just buried his dad in January of that same year.

Approximately ten days later, my gynecologist's office called for me to come in as soon as possible to speak with Dr. B. about the pathology report from the exploratory surgery. I was a little confused. It was then I learned that anything that is removed from the body goes to pathology. The infected stitch apparently had cancerous cells attached to it. Dr B. was suddenly referring me to an oncologist to discuss treatment and a plan of action. I had uterine cancer with metastatic cells near my bladder. Words like early stage, margins, grade, blood work, cell counts, and labs all went past my mind. My ears seemed muffled and I knew I was sitting in the chair but I didn't feel present at all. Did she tell me that I had cancer? I was already taking care of my elderly mother (Mama "A") at home who had recently gone into remission from colon cancer. This wasn't happening. But it was.

Meeting with the oncologist was surreal. I liked Dr. R. a lot and she took her time explaining all the different terms and abbreviations that were now going to be a part of my daily vocabulary. I was scheduled for eight rounds of radiation therapy (one round is five days, 20 minutes each day). After radiation I would then begin six rounds of chemotherapy. With this new information, I met with my radiologist and did my preparation for my first radiation treatment. The tech measured and then drew specific lines on my abdomen with a sharpie. It was a big area and looked like a map. I was instructed to not wash it off or swim and to show up at 10:20 every morning at oncology for treatment. The nurse handed me my oncology parking pass and I was on my way.

It was Father's Day weekend and we were spending it by the pool. Treatment would start on Monday. It was the first Father's Day my hubby would be without his dad. Our daughter also brought her new boyfriend to the house for us to meet him. There were lots of feelings going on inside of me. Our daughter began introducing her boyfriend to us. When it was my turn, she said, "And this is my stepmom. She likes to write on herself with markers." Humor is always my go to. I'm glad I have a humorous family. Incidentally, I did go swimming that day.

Monday morning I found myself in the oncology parking lot. I remembered being here every day when I would bring my mum for her treatments. I could feel the anxiety starting to surface. I prayed. I threw the parking pass away on my way inside. I refused to enter through the oncology doors so I entered through the main entrance of the hospital and walked a maze to radiation. Everyone was really nice. I got on the table, laid flat on my back and was told to remain very still.

I took a deep breath and prayed some more. The machine resembled the back of a huge concrete truck and was being directed over top of me. I wondered if I would smell burning skin. I didn't and it was painless. At least for now. This part was just the beginning. I still remembered my mum's side effects all too clearly.

I finished all eight rounds of radiation but had to take some breaks in between due to the burning of my skin. It felt like I was sunburned badly on the inside and out. There were several large oozing blisters and my skin was peeling off all around my abdomen and lady parts. It was very painful. I was constantly exhausted and sleep was always interrupted anytime fabric touched my burnt skin. I was relieved to have the radiation behind me. Next step would be chemotherapy.

I started out at home taking doses of cyclophosphamide via pill form. The day I picked up the prescription from the pharmacy I rode around with it in my purse for a few hours. Next thing I knew, I was in a store wandering around and on the phone with my husband. He gently calmed me down while I freaked out about the fact that I was about to start poisoning myself voluntarily. How do you even begin to console someone in this situation? But he did, just like always. I did the dance with the cyclophosphamide for several weeks off and on. Some of my hair fell out but I was able to mask it pretty well since I have the thickest hair in the world. I noticed a queasiness that became a constant along with never ending fatigue. It was very similar to having the flu. I had multiple medications prescribed for the many side effects from chemo. Those prescription drugs came with a list of their own side effects. I didn't have the stamina I used to yet I still continued to work and stay in denial as much as possible. By the end of my last round of chemo, I was sent along my merry way with a clean bill of health and checkups every 3 months. It takes a very long time for chemo to get out of your body and awhile before you regain strength again.

I made it almost a year before I had the second recurrence of cancer. I had been horseback riding with my girlfriends. It was cold that day and I was tired. We had such a great time. Next thing I remember, my husband and daughter were picking me up as I was lying face down on the floor half in and half out of the garage. Needless to say, it scared them both but I convinced them

I was fine and probably needed to eat something. I knew I wasn't fine. I had never passed out before.

That week I was in my doctor's office getting labs pulled and without hesitation my doctor immediately began ordering multiple tests. My white cells had depleted tremendously and it was possible that I now had leukemia. There was that muffled feeling in my ears again.

The MRI showed a mass in my abdominal area with two tiny spots on my lower spine. Good news, not leukemia. Instead, it was peritoneal cancer (also treated like ovarian cancer). My oncologist scheduled me for more chemotherapy. This treatment would be via infusion. Dr. R explained that I would first be scheduled for a surgical procedure to put a port into my chest that the chemo would be a administered through. I remembered my Mama "A" having to do this. I could feel a panic attack washing over me and began to pray scattered prayers silently to God. Dr. R explained that a chemo cocktail would be prescribed to treat this type of cancer. A cocktail is several types of chemotherapy drugs that you get at one time. Mine were to be Taxol, Cyclophosphamide and Methotrexate. I learned quickly that these were not friendly. As the appointment came to a close, I knew the plan of attack, but wasn't at peace about the port going in and against Dr. R's advice, I declined, which meant the chemo would be infused into a vein in my arm or neck. This was how I chose to do things. Dr. R and I were not off to a good start this time around.

Six long, miserable and grueling rounds of chemo came and went. I had black and blue arms and neck from multiple needle punctures and collapsed veins. Each round was worse than the last. I never knew a person could vomit so much in a lifetime.

Some days it was both ends. Other days I would dry heave until my ears rang, or blood vessels popped in my eyes and I would swear I wasn't going to be able to catch my next breath. The chills, the hot flashes, the headaches, the deep bone pain—the horrific chemo sores in my mouth, throat, nose and genitals--it was all terrible. Nausea medications were given but my body didn't respond to them. I blew up from the steroids that were in my chemo cocktail. The nausea was so bad that I even had a travel neck pillow that I would set on the toilet seat to lie my face on when I couldn't hold my head up anymore to puke. Some days I thought I wanted to die. During one of those days, my daughter came home from a date with her guy. She stood outside the bathroom door telling me bits and pieces of her evening but the thing that I will always remember most is when she told me with sweet excitement that he had told her he loved her for the very first time. She knew I was puking my guts out but it didn't stop normal life events. I may have been knocked to the ground from cancer, but cancer wasn't robbing us of our special moments. We functioned well considering the circumstances—or so I convinced myself.

My husband bought a Harley and as sick as I was, I would hurl my big leg over that bike, hold onto "my old man" (that's HOG talk) and ride for miles. I used to fall asleep on the back of the bike and my hubby would frequently tap my legs to keep me alert. I even learned how to vomit off the back of the bike without stopping or getting any of it on us or the bike. You get over your phobia of public restrooms quickly when you're on chemo. Our family rode dirt bikes together, too. We all had one.

I wiped out most of the time (I really just wanted to bond with and impress my young teenage son) but they never discouraged me from trying to live and have fun. Your mental thinking and your attitude play such a big part in any battle in your life.

Another blow came when my comfort of all comforts had to be put to sleep two days before Christmas. That did me in. I had come home from treatment and spent the last moments I had cuddling with my sweet boy, Cody. He was a Golden Retriever/Cocker Spaniel mix. He was considered to be a mutt when we found each other at the local SPCA, but today that mix of breeds are called Comfort Retrievers and they sell for up to $1,500.00 a pup! But a comfort he was as we held each other closely for those last moments together. At 3:00 pm our vet was kind enough to make a house call and allow us to be in the comfort of our home for the procedure. My husband and I sobbed uncontrollably and another part of me died on that day. Christmas sucked.

By the end of my sixth round of chemo, I had become septic and anemic. Twice I cried and begged and pleaded to not be admitted to the hospital. Instead, I was sent home and could sleep for days at a time. I had multiple types of medications and somewhere during all of this, Mama "A" formed a blood clot in her leg and fell at home. I, in turn, lifted her off the floor and blew out my back, landing us both in separate ambulance rides to the hospital. Mama "A" was on the first floor and I was on the second and my husband was losing his mind.

Ephesians 6:10-18 The Armor of God

Finally, be strong in the Lord and in his mighty power. Put on the full armor of God, so that you can take your stand against the devil's schemes. For our struggle is not against flesh and blood, but against the rulers, against the authorities, against the powers of this dark world and against the spiritual forces of evil in the heavenly realms. Therefore put on the full armor of God, so that when the day of evil comes, you may be able to stand your ground, and after you have done everything, to stand. Stand firm then, with the belt of truth buckled around your waist, with the breastplate of righteousness in place, and with your feet fitted with the readiness that comes from the gospel of peace. In addition to all this, take up the shield of faith, with which you can extinguish all the flaming arrows of the evil one. Take the helmet of salvation and the sword of the Spirit, which is the word of God.

By 2011 I had a brief celebration with a clean and clear bill of health but within a few short months I had another recurrence with the "C" beast. This time the mass was attacking my spine and appeared to be aggressive. More chemotherapy treatments were immediately set up and three more rounds of radiation. I wanted to scream bloody murder. I was irate and scared and furious and so damn disappointed. It wasn't fair.

My Mama "A" was now in a long term nursing care facility. My husband had to make that judgment call because I was so loaded out of my mind on multiple painkillers (the three D's: Dilaudid, Demerol, and Darvocet) and opioid drugs (Oxycotin, Oxycodone, Valium, Fentanyl) that I wasn't mentally present for about three months. Weaning off of these types of drugs can throw your mental balance and physical balance into a chemical train wreck. I was thrown into a pit of depression and despair that was life- threatening. I cried, hid under the covers, became reclusive and shut out my friends and relatives. I learned how to shop online, and navigate through social media. This was how I socialized since I was too ill to be around others due to my depleted immune system. Cancer was determined to steal everything.

Our daughter was preparing to leave for college. She and I had been packing for a couple of days trying to make everything fit into the vehicles. Tensions were high from nerves and stress. It was late morning when my husband came home and announced that after 17 years of employment, he no longer had a job. The economy tanked. We were both now currently unemployed. The next day, we drove our girl to JMU.

This next chemo experience came via infusion into the base of my spinal cord as to attack the mass more directly. Two infusions were also administered rectally. The treatment took 6 to 7 hours and I didn't get to sit amongst the other patients I had become acquainted with because I was in an isolated room laying on my side or stomach. These were the treatments that were killing me. My body wasn't strong enough to endure the amount of poison being pumped into it. My bones were excruciating with pain and the chemo headaches were like nothing I can explain. My hair was falling out, again, and so my husband shaved my head in the middle of the kitchen as we both cried.

During this third encounter with chemo I was beyond weak. I was forced to quit my job after just returning back to it and couldn't get rid of the nausea and vomiting. I would cry, cradling my head from the multiple chemo headaches, and on a whim became desperate enough to try something a few of my fellow cancer buddies were doing. Something that I was deeply against.

Genesis 1:29-31 (NIV) 29 Then God said "I give you every seed-bearing plant on the face of the whole earth and every tree that has fruit with seed in it. They will be yours for food. 30 And to all the beasts of the earth and all the birds in the sky and all the creatures that move along the ground-everything that has the breath of life in it-I give every green plant for food." And it was so.

31 God saw all that he had made and it was very good. And there was evening, and there was morning--the sixth day.

My husband is an amazing man. I tell him he is all my movie channels because he really is. When it came time to act on the decision based on pure desperation, my husband left the house and was back within 20 minutes rolling a blunt for the first time in 20+ years. He claimed he didn't do a bad job considering it had been so long. I remembered trying marijuana a couple of times in high school but never liked it or had a need to explore further. I took the joint, lit the end and inhaled some of it into my lungs. Nothing. I still felt like I had been run over by a train. I had another puff, coughed and choked and not long after, felt a sensational feeling of pure relaxation. Any painful areas just became hot. The nausea subsided and anything my hubby said or did made me laugh hysterically. I love to laugh. I actually felt kind of good for the first time in years. I also got the munchies. I was able to eat again and hold the food down when I smoked. I still had the metallic taste in my mouth from the chemo but this cannabis was actually helping me feel better.

For awhile I was afraid of it. I wasn't educated about cannabis and as a Christian, struggled tremendously with myself that I was sinning and/or doing something illegal. It's a difficult situation to find yourself in. It wasn't the high I wanted but the relief, the instant relief it brought to my battered body. It wasn't long before I started dumping the anti-nausea drugs and painkillers from my regimen. I actually felt pretty darn good. In November, I brought home a three month old Golden Retriever puppy and named him, Sunny. We bonded instantly and he helped to fill the void I had now that our daughter was gone. Day-by-day, we faced what came our way. My husband struggled to find a new job that could maintain our current expenses. Our health insurance for a family of four was over $2,000.00 per month and my out-of-pocket medical expenses were accumulating uncontrollably. The struggle was real and we kept clinging to our faith.

We made our way into another summer when it became evident that my body simply could not endure anymore chemo or radiation. I was saturated. I was due for a PET scan which showed very little improvement. The peritoneal lining was now showing another mass and with no more chemo my outlook would be 12 to 14 months of maybe quality life. There was that muffled silence again and this time I already felt dead. *Alright, God,* I thought. *This is it.* The only thing left was chemotherapy for what was left of the duration on my life but my body was shutting down slowly because of it. Either cancer or the treatments were going to take me. I left my oncologist and drove to the beach. I got out of my car and sat on the sand staring at the beautiful ocean and all its power. I prayed but I was numb. Moments later, my movie channel man sat down beside me, held me close and we didn't utter a word. It was time to get my affairs in order.

Music is a very important part of my daily life. I must have it and I love many genres. My sweet friend, Marsh-MEL-ow, gifted me with a wonderful IPod and set of BOSE headphones that were (and still are) one of my saving graces. I had assorted "chemo" playlists for the days I had chemo. Some days during treatments I listened to praise and worship and other days uplifting, pop music about strength and survival. There was a playlist with what I refer to as "angry man" music that sings about dying and being pissed off. Other times I listened to calming spa music, motivational preaching and my most favorite of all, Reggae. I had music for any and all moods. As I sat adding more songs to playlists, someone I love dearly came and handed me a syringe which contained a dark, thick, sticky substance. This substance was actually made from cannabis and is also known as RSO oil. I recommend researching this if you are interested in alternative medicine or treatments. This oil contains a very high THC content and is believed to actually fight existing cancer cells. This oil was also obtained at great lengths and high risks by someone who loved their spouse deeply enough to risk their own life. They were loving, kind, gracious and generous enough to give us this oil in hope of a miracle. They too were fighting the cancer battle and many of my cancer buddies were dying all around me. It will leave you with survivor's guilt.

I began taking the oil. Small amounts over the course of several hours until you slowly build a tolerance to the side effects. With research and helpful resources I began educating myself more and more about this sticky, greasy oil. I noticed that it had challenging side effects at first, mostly fatigue. I slept and slept. When it was time to meet with my oncologist I told her that I was throwing in the towel with anymore chemo. I wanted to give this oil a shot. This decision was not at all encouraged and my doctor's reaction was abrupt. I was extremely disappointed. Although my doctor was only advising me as to what she believed to be the surest way to continue treatment, we couldn't seem to agree to disagree. I continued with the oil on my own for the next four months. I slowly increased the dosage that I had researched online. I continued having my lab work done and miraculously, my depleted blood cell counts were climbing with great results. Symptoms from the chemo and radiation were slowly dissipating. I took the oil for four months before it was time for my next PET scan. The results of this PET scan were phenomenal. Only a tiny spot near the spine remained and it was recorded as scar tissue because of its minimal size. For the first time in eight years I heard the words, "No evidence of cancer" (NEC). Praise God!

Currently, I am over two years cancer free. I continue on a maintenance dose of the cannabis oil. I also use essential oils and pay attention to my diet. Exercise is minimal due to the severe damage to my lower spine from the chemo and radiation treatments. I am able to swim as a means of therapy and have had multiple stem cell procedures to try and rebuild the damaged bone and tissue in my lower back. Chemo brain is still present and I forget things in an instant. I get about four or five hours out of a day before I have to sleep and recharge my body. I still hurt and sometimes have nausea or tingling in my lower body. It hurts to sit or stand for any great length of time. I'm unable to return to a full time job.

What I am, however, is grateful. I'm alive and I'm getting stronger. I do believe that chemo and radiation treatments did carry me through phases of my journey with cancer but it also wreaked havoc in my body and I learned how important it is to explore all the options that you can. Be diligent and never ever be afraid to speak up or ask questions. You have to become your own advocate.

We were forced to sell our dream home in 2016. It devastated me at first. We were beaten down and exhausted. Mama "A" passed away in February of 2015 at the age of 92 from colon cancer. Our daughter married that great guy who is now our son-in-love and our son joined the Navy and is serving this great country proudly. Mama "B" is now fighting for her life with stage 4 colon cancer. My movie channel man is finally getting to breathe and have fun. We have new plans and ideas for our future. I've learned that less is more. I love harder and deeper and appreciate the smallest things.

I love God with all my heart and it is important for me to share how in love God is with you. He will never force himself onto you. God is a gentleman and once He is invited, He will show Himself mightily. Your life could not be better. Hang out with him. Call on Him. Know Him. I promise you won't regret it. I could not have survived this journey without Him.

"For God so loved the world that he gave his one and only Son, that whoever believes in him shall not perish but have eternal life" (John 3:16).

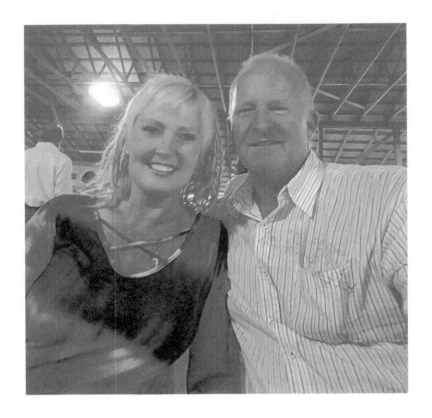

Susie & Tommy

STUDY GUIDE

This section of the book is designed to help our readers ponder some of the universal questions that emerge in our story. Whether you take time alone to process the following questions or go through the book with a group or club, we encourage you to face each chapter and question withtheutmostauthenticityand honesty. Most importantly, as you work through the study guide, remember that you are not alone!

Chapter One:

Chapter one introduces us to Andrea and Lenny on the day Lenny was first diagnosed with Non-Hodgkins Lymphoma. By the end of the chapter, we understand that the journey we are about to embark on with them has proven to be the most difficult of their marriage and their lives. There are many things that can happen in life that are completely out of our control, and we can choose to allow life's disappointments make us bitter or make us better. Andrea shares that in retrospect, she can see how the journey they traveled has made them better.

How do you handle life's unexpected tragedies and obstacles when they hit?

What has retrospect taught you about yourself and the way you deal with the unexpected?

Do you wish you dealt with difficult things differently?

If so, in what way?

Chapter Two:

In chapter two we discover that Lenny's prognosis is to watch and wait. Through the process of learning more about the cancer and the treatment options available to him, Lenny and Andrea realize that they aren't willing to take this news sitting down. They will fight to find a solution for Lenny's health. Because of an experience in Andrea's past, she has confidence in methods other than those available through traditional physicians. Even though they don't understand why they are on this path, they are determined to do all they can to find healing.

What obstacles are you facing that seem impossible or without a solution?

Who can you turn to for guidance, strength, or inspiration in facing these obstacles?

Chapter Three:

Chapter three takes us into the world of alternative medicine and the series of doubts, conflicting emotions, and ultimate victories that comes with choosing a path that is controversial and unknown. By the end we understand that there is a vast difference between the alternative medical world and conventional medicine as Andrea and Lenny face the realization that not all of their progress will be seen as such by conventional doctors. Instead, they fight to stay positive and receive positive reinforcement from the medical world.

How do you respond to those who don't support your endeavors or provide positive feedback to your goals and accomplishments?

Who in your life do you trust to stand with you and provide encouragement in the face of either an obstacle or challenge?

What alternative options have you researched (If applicable) to help you overcome your obstacles?

Chapter Four:

Chapter four reveals the tragic loss of two babies that Andrea and Lenny faced in the midst of their fight for Lenny's life. We also discover that Andrea and Lenny are believers and approach their daily lives with faith in Christ. Through their story, we begin to see that while they face life with an incredible determination and strength, the many challenges thrown their way are also causing an underlying brokenness that is difficult to face—or fix—in the midst of the battle with cancer.

How does your belief system influence the way you face challenges in life?

What past experiences, if any, still feel raw or painful to think about?

Take time to process any experiences that come to mind. Is there anyone you need to forgive, including yourself?

How can you open your heart to find healing from those experiences? Take time to pray and ask God to heal any wounds that remain.

Chapter Five:

In chapter five, Lenny and Andrea are faced with the scary question of time and not knowing how much time they have left together as a family. As they face this reality, they begin to ask difficult questions and realize that the most important thing they can do is live life to the fullest. In the midst of this realization, they experience the beauty of generosity and help from those around them, as well as the inspiration of new life in the arrival of their son Jordan. Life and death are inevitable and because God gives us all free will, we must choose how we do both wisely.

How were you impacted by the question that Lenny faces in this chapter: Now that you might die, how will you choose to live?

If time were of the essence, what things would you want to see, do or accomplish in the time remaining?

In what ways did this chapter challenge your perspective on life, time, family and death?

Chapter Six:

Chapter six chronicles the decision that Andrea and Lenny make to go through conventional treatment. Because his cancer has influenced other parts of his body, Lenny is faced with the decision to get chemo and radiation to stop the spread of the cancer cells. Andrea and Lenny experience an internal struggle of choosing treatment while knowing that it is also damaging Lenny's body.

When have you faced a decision that seemingly conflicts with your beliefs or convictions?

How did you make your decision in the midst of the conflict? What was your process?

What did that experience (or experiences) teach you about yourself and your beliefs?

Chapter Seven:

In this chapter, we learn more about Lenny and his strategy for getting through chemotherapy treatments. In his determination to get through to the other side, he mentally challenges himself to fight the good fight and check of each day, one at a time. He discovers how to not take his life for granted and he also finds that his will to live is tied to his desire to raise his children and be there for them as they grow up.

What moments or experiences have challenged you to not take life for granted?

In the midst of struggle, what things—both internal and external—motivate you to keep going?

What did you learn or realize through Lenny's story of fighting the good fight?

Chapter Eight:

Chapter Eight brings us closer to Andrea and her struggle with depression throughout her life and particularly during the years she acted as caregiver to her husband. In the midst of her journey, she learns the importance of asking for help, the grace that comes from her relationship with God, and the priceless gift that comes in the form of unsolicited support from friends and strangers. Whether or not we ourselves struggle with depression, this chapter challenges us to look at the world, and those around us, through different eyes and with a heart to love.

Do you struggle with asking for help from those around you? How can you challenge yourself to both seek and accept help this week?

What is one practical thing you can do for someone in need this week?

Is there anyone in your life who may be struggling more than you realized? How can you provide support for them during this time?

Chapter Nine:

Chapter nine is about facing the unknown and how even something as desired as remission is filled with unknowns. Lenny and Andrea walk through a series of losses: the real estate crash, the loss of jobs, their home and eventually both of their fathers. While struggling to walk through these losses, they also must make decisions about life without having a plan, a contingency, or a clue about what lies ahead.

When have you been faced with a life decision, big or small, in the midst of the unknown?

What or who helped you make decisions and move forward despite not knowing if you were making the right decision?

How would you encourage yourself and others in the midst of the unknown?

Chapter Ten:

In chapter ten, Lenny is once again faced with the conflicting decision to receive conventional treatment. Even in the midst of choosing chemo and a stem cell transplant, Lenny decides he wants to continue pursuing alternative options. After his transplant, Andrea embarks on a journey to make cannabis oil, a potential treatment option. It is here that we fully understand that it is her love for Lenny that has been the driving force behind the entire endeavor toward healing. We also come to learn that walking in peace is a continuous journey of the soul and one that is tested in the midst of trials.

3 John 2 is referenced in this chapter: "Beloved, I pray that you may prosper in all things and be in health, just as your soul prospers." What does this verse mean to you?

What does it look like for your soul to prosper or be at peace? How do you find peace in the midst of life's many challenges?

Chapter Eleven:

Chapter eleven introduces us to the clinic in Mexico and a part of Lenny's healing journey when he and Andrea find rest and revelation about the years of choices, challenges, and uncertainty. Lenny and Andrea find themselves surrounded by people who are both encouraging and in need of encouragement, and they realize that what they desire most is to share their love and their knowledge with those in need.

What would life look like if you were constantly surrounded by people who love, support and encourage you in all that you do?

Are there people in your life who you can invest in to both bring encouragement and receive encouragement from them?

What is one thing you can do or say today to show someone your support and encouragement?

Chapter Twelve:

Chapter twelve brings us back to the United States and shows us how Lenny and Andrea choose to implement their new knowledge and their renewed conviction that alternative medicine adds value to people's health and well being. They realize that everything they have tried or attempted has helped Lenny's health improve in one way or another. They also learn to walk in complete peace with their decisions and convictions in spite of criticism or hesitancy from the conventional medical world.

In what ways has your hope for a certain outcome ever been challenged or threatened?

What have you done to maintain both peace and hope in the midst of those challenging circumstances?

Take a moment to consider areas of your life where you need renewed hope. Ask God to show you His perspective about those areas of your life.

Chapter Thirteen:

Chapter thirteen reveals the beauty of love and the gift that has been in Andrea and Lenny's lives. Without their faith in God, without the love of Christ and the love of other people, they would not be standing in victory today. It is through God's grace and goodness that they have been able to fight, to keep going, and to provide love and support to other people along the way.

How has love influenced your life in a positive way?

Andrea writes, "When we understand our worth, our place in this world and the unique value we bring to it—we suddenly have a purpose to keep fighting." What is your purpose or the unique value that you bring to the world?

If you struggled with the above question, take a moment to ask God what your unique purpose is on this earth.

How does your experience of love motivate you to share that love with others? What does that look like?

What one thing can you do this week to demonstrate love to those around you?

ABOUT THE AUTHORS

Andrea's journey and passion with health, wellness, and a love for helping others began over 20 years ago. An accomplished real estate agent in Virginia, she has served hundreds of clients in building, reselling and acquiring the home of their dreams. It was early on in her real estate career when she met the love of her life, Lenny London.

Together they built a strong faith-based family and love for helping others. While working with several health companies, in pursuit of a deeper knowledge and for the family's optimal health, Andrea realized her new passion for motivating others toward a healthier lifestyle and sharing God's message of love with the world.

When Lenny developed cancer in December of 2001, their pursuit for alternative healing for the mind, body and spirit was solidified and a new mission was formed. Their life experience of finding different roads toward healing and prevention for Lenny and motivating others toward great health inspired them to want to educate others and make a positive impact. Today, Andrea shares these life experiences through various forms of media and speaking engagements.

Andrea & Lenny reside in Virginia Beach and have four children, Blake, Diana, Dylan & Jordan. They work toward creating a Wellness Ministry which will assist in sending people battling cancer to alternative places of healing including clinics in Mexico where Lenny had incredible success.